Attention-Deficit Hyperactivity Disorder (ADHD) in Adults

Key Issues in Mental Health

Vol. 176

Series Editors

A. Riecher-Rössler Basel

M. Steiner Hamilton

Attention-Deficit Hyperactivity Disorder (ADHD) in Adults

Volume Editors

Wolfgang Retz Homburg/Saar

Rachel G. Klein New York, N.Y.

9 figures and 18 tables, 2010

KARGER

Basel · Freiburg · Paris · London · New York · Bangalore · Bangkok · Shanghai · Singapore · Tokyo · Sydney

Key Issues in Mental Health
Formerly published as 'Bibliotheca Psychiatrica' (founded 1917)

Prof. Dr. Wolfgang Retz
Institut für Gerichtliche
Psychologie und Psychiatrie
Universitätskliniken des
Saarlandes
Kirrberger Strasse
Homburg/Saar (Germany)

Rachel G. Klein, MD
Department of Child and
Adolescent Psychiatry
New York University
Child Study Center
New York, N.Y. (USA)

Library of Congress Cataloging-in-Publication Data

Attention-deficit hyperactivity disorder (ADHD) in adults / volume editors,
Wolfgang Retz, Rachel G. Klein.
p. ; cm. -- (Key issues in mental health, ISSN 1662-4874; v. 176)
Includes bibliographical references and indexes.
ISBN 978-3-8055-9237-6 (hardcover : alk. paper)
1. Attention-deficit disorder in adults. I. Retz, Wolfgang. II. Klein,
Rachel G. III. Series: Key issues in mental health, v. 176. 1662-4874;
[DNLM: 1. Attention-Deficit Disorder with Hyperactivity--diagnosis. 2.
Adult. 3. Attention-Deficit Disorder with Hyperactivity--therapy. W1 BI429
v.176 / WM 190 A883 2010]
RC394.A85A884 2010
616.85'89--dc22

2009037557

Bibliographic Indices. This publication is listed in bibliographic services, including Current Contents®

www.karger.com
Printed in Switzerland on acid-free and non-aging paper (ISO 9706) by Reinhardt Druck, Basel
ISSN 1662–4874
ISBN 978–3–8055–9237–6
e-ISBN 978–3–8055–9238–3

Contents

Preface

Despite a long research history and robust findings about genetics, life course, and treatment of attention-deficit hyperactivity disorder (ADHD), the disorder remains a matter of public controversies and scientific debates. Descriptions of children suffering from developmentally inadequate inattention, motor overactivity and impulsivity by European as well as American physicians go back to the 19th century. In the 20th century, empirical studies across the world substantially advanced our knowledge of epidemiology, etiology, pathophysiology and treatment of the syndrome. Nevertheless, controversy about the diagnosis remains, as evidenced by different diagnostic standards in the Diagnostic and Statistical Manual of the American Psychiatric Association (4th ed.; DSM-IV), and the International Classification of Diseases (10th ed.; ICD-10), which is more restrictive and is the obligatory diagnostic standard for European psychiatrists. Due to the immense international scientific support for the DSM-IV approach to the diagnosis of ADHD, it is applied in this volume of *Key Issues in Mental Health*.

Although disbelieved for many decades, longitudinal studies performed since the 1970s in the USA, Canada and other countries have clearly shown that ADHD persists into adulthood and is associated with high risk for comorbid psychiatric disorders and social impairment. Until recently, in Germany and other European countries, the lifespan perspective of this disorder has failed to be recognized. In the last decade, scientific and clinical interest in ADHD have increased dramatically in Germany, but there remains a deep transatlantic gap regarding treatment opportunities, and views about the benefits of treatment, for adult ADHD patients, in spite of ample empirical evidence supporting treatment efficacy.

In this volume of *Key Issues in Mental Health*, we have brought together scientists from the USA and Germany to provide an overview about several important aspects of ADHD across the lifespan. The topics include epidemiology, neurobiology, psychopathology, longitudinal course, comorbidity and social impairment. Moreover, diagnostic problems and therapeutic options regarding this disorder are discussed.

In the first chapter, Paul H. Wender and David A. Tomb give a synopsis of adult ADHD from the authors' extended work at the University of Utah. Formal and molecular genetic studies are reviewed by Christine M. Freitag and Wolfgang Retz in chapters 2 and 3, followed by chapter 4, where Christina G. Baehne and Andreas J. Fallgatter report findings from neurophysiological studies of adult ADHD. An overview of morphological and functional imaging studies in adult ADHD is provided by Marc Schneider and coworkers in chapter 5. The subsequent chapters refer to clinical aspects of ADHD in adults, starting with diagnostic issues of adult ADHD, presented in chapter 6 by Rolf-Dieter Stieglitz. The very important issue of comorbidity in adult ADHD is reviewed by Rachel G. Klein and Salvatore Mannuzza in chapter 7, and in chapter 8 aspects of social dysfunctioning in adults with ADHD are discussed by Michael Rösler. The last two chapters give insights into therapeutic approaches in adult ADHD. In chapter 9, Alexandra Philipsen and coworkers report on psychotherapeutic approaches for adults with ADHD, with a main focus on the development of a group therapy in Germany, and in chapter 10 Götz-Erik Trott summarizes options of pharmacological treatment.

In order to continue the tradition of *Key Issues in Mental Health*, the editors and contributing authors endeavored to give an overview of the most relevant research and treatments in an important field of contemporary psychiatry. We hope that this volume will be a useful tool for physicians and therapists who work with ADHD patients.

Wolfgang Retz
Rachel G. Klein

Chapter 1

Retz W, Klein RG (eds): Attention-Deficit Hyperactivity Disorder (ADHD) in Adults.
Key Issues in Mental Health. Basel, Karger, 2010, vol 176, pp 1–37

Attention-Deficit Hyperactivity Disorder in Adults: An Overview

Paul H. Wender[a] · David A. Tomb[b]

[a]Department of Psychiatry, Harvard Medical School, Boston, Mass., and [b]Department of Psychiatry, University of Utah School of Medicine, Salt Lake City, Utah, USA

Abstract

Attention-deficit hyperactivity disorder (ADHD) is a common, genetically transmitted neurological disorder, with onset in childhood, probably mediated in part by decreased brain dopaminergic functioning. The first author and colleagues were among the earliest (1976) to describe the persistence of symptoms into adulthood and to perform a methylphenidate trial. Prevalence and natural history data suggest that of the 3–10% of children diagnosed with ADHD, one- to two-thirds continue to manifest appreciable ADHD symptoms as adults. This chapter reviews how ADHD in adults can be readily diagnosed and treated using the Wender Utah diagnostic criteria to identify adult characteristics of the disorder. Stringent diagnosis is key to determining effective treatment. This chapter also addresses core hypotheses of etiology and treatment. Dopamine agonist stimulant medications appear to be the most effective in treating ADHD. About 70% of patients receiving stimulant medication have shown moderate to marked improvement, as compared with 20% of those receiving placebo. The core symptoms of hyperactivity, inattention, mood lability, temper, disorganization, stress sensitivity, and impulsivity have been shown to respond to treatment with stimulant medications more than to other drugs. Appropriate management of adult patients with ADHD includes psychoeducation and counseling when necessary while the roles of supportive problem-directed therapy, behavioral intervention, coaching, and couples and family therapy remain to be evaluated.

Attention-deficit hyperactivity disorder (ADHD) is very likely the most common and undiagnosed psychiatric disorder of adult life. Increasingly recognized only since the 1970s, ADHD had previously been believed to diminish in adolescence and disappear in adulthood. About 30 years ago, the senior author noted that the parents of ADHD children described similar problems in their own childhood and for many these problems had continued throughout life. A frequent comment by a spouse was: 'What do you mean used to have?' The senior author was then faced with two primary questions: [1] what clinical features characterize ADHD in adults (this work antedated DSM-III) and [2] how does one determine if the adults would have met the criteria for ADHD as children since it is believed that the condition does not appear de novo in adulthood.

With a focus on adults, this chapter outlines the history of the diagnostic concept, its prevalence, clinical medical symptoms, diagnosis and differential diagnosis, presumed etiology and (briefly) treatment. Much of this is based on 30 years of work conducted by Wender and colleagues and their efforts to clarify the two essential questions above. The interested reader is referred to his recent review article or book *Attention-Deficit Hyperactivity Disorder in Adults* for more detail [1, 2].

History of the ADHD Concept

The names and criteria for the syndrome of ADHD have changed frequently. What is now referred to as ADHD has been variously designated as 'minimal brain damage', 'minimal brain dysfunction', 'minimal cerebral dysfunction', 'hyperkinesis', and the 'hyperactive child syndrome'. The main behavioral and/or cognitive abnormalities contained within the syndrome usually included overactivity, inattentiveness, impulsivity, affective lability and 'immaturity'. Associated abnormalities included, but were not limited to, poor peer relations, defiance, hostility, 'acting out' behaviors and 'learning problems'. The earliest descriptions of a behavioral condition akin to ADHD were provided by George Still at the turn of the century [3]. He posited an overarching failure in moral control and proposed a biological substrate (either hereditary and/or the result of some acquired encephalopathy). His formulation of underlying CNS damage was reflected in the early diagnostic terms of minimal brain damage or minimal brain dysfunction (both MBD), which prevailed throughout the first half of the 20th century.

Subsequent conceptual shifts are reflected in the several versions of the *Diagnostic and Statistical Manual of Mental Disorders* (DSM) published by the American Psychiatric Association. A more descriptive view was taken in 1968 such that the second edition called the disorder Hyperkinetic Reaction of Childhood, and stressed abnormally high levels of motor activity as the primary deficit. Later research emphasized deficits in attention and impulse control, as well as hyperactivity [4]. Consequently in 1980 the third revision of the DSM (DSM-III) re-titled it Attention Deficit Disorder (ADD), with two subtypes (with or without hyperactivity) [5]. Debates continued as to the central importance of problems with hyperactivity, and in 1987 the disorder was renamed Attention Deficit/Hyperactivity Disorder (DSM-III-R). ADD without hyperactivity was named Undifferentiated Attention Deficit Disorder, and thought by many to embody a separate disorder of attention [6–8]. The most current DSM-IV (1994) melds the different emphases by titling the disorder ADHD/Primarily Inattentive Type, or ADHD/Primarily Hyperactive-Impulsive Type, or ADHD/Combined Type, depending on the mix of inattentive, hyperactive or impulsive symptoms [9].

All of the above terminology reflects evolving theories of etiology or key symptoms. Future advances in understanding the biology and pathophysiology of the disorder may yet lead us to further nosological shifts [see, for example, Retz and Freitag, Baehne and Fallgatter, and Schneider et al., chapters 3, 4 and 5].

Core Symptoms

Although a former version of the DSM included the category of 'ADHD-residual type', there are no specific criteria for ADHD in adults. The DSM-IV's symptomatic criteria were developed for children and, not surprisingly, many of them are age-limited and look exclusively at behavior. In this category are behaviors such as 'often runs about or climbs excessively...' or 'often has difficulty playing or engaging in leisure activities quietly'. These criteria are not applicable to adulthood, which makes defining relevant and age-appropriate symptoms a critical issue. Versions of DSM-III (1980–1994) upon which much research has been based was even more inappropriate by using descriptions such as: 'has difficulty waiting turn in games or group situations.' Moreover, the DSM criteria focus on only three symptoms/behaviors of adult ADHD: inattention, hyperactivity, and impulsivity. There is no effort to assess the variety of broader problems that appear to accompany ADHD in adults. Accordingly, since 1976, the senior author has been developing tentative operational criteria for ADHD in an attempt to better specify characteristics more directly relevant to adults.

Childhood Status

By definition, ADHD begins in childhood. Thus the first task of the clinician is to determine the psychiatric status of the patient as a child and to make a retrospective diagnosis of childhood ADHD. Some patients may have been evaluated or treated as children. For others we inquire about the presence or absence of DSM-IV ADHD symptoms during childhood. However, many ADHD adults' memories of their childhood are cloudy and inaccurate and we lack a measure of reliability. In 2002, Mannuzza interviewed ADHD subjects and controls as children and then again about their childhood symptoms when they were adults and found that retrospective diagnoses of ADHD in childhood, based on the subjects' adult memories, were inaccurate in 73% of cases. As a screening procedure one can seek to obtain a history of the more macro (and presumably better recalled) behavioral characterizations (see below). To further circumvent a memory problem we have also employed the three approaches outlined below. Parental interview is the first and preferred method of obtaining childhood symptoms. If this is not possible, a useful second approach is for the patient's parents to rate their (now) adult offspring as he or she had been in childhood, using the 'Parents Rating Scale' (PRS) (see appendix A). The PRS is a

10-item adaptation of the Conner's Rating Scale popularly used for childhood ADHD assessment, and yields an index of the magnitude of an adult's hyperactivity during childhood [10]. The PRS has been normed and a score of 12 or greater (0–3/item) places the adult patient in the 95th percentile for childhood 'hyperactivity' within the United States population. Other populations will require further standardization. The third technique is to administer the Wender Utah Rating Scale (WURS). It is a patient self-rating scale for childhood behavior and symptoms of 61 items consistent with ADHD/Combined Type (see appendix B).

The 25 most discriminating items are scored in a 0–4 rating scale [11]. This scale has been standardized in normal adults, adults with a major depressive disorder, and adults with ADHD and has been translated into and standardized in German [12].

Utah Criteria

The senior author and his collaborators have developed a set of characteristics to specify both necessary childhood criteria and current ADHD symptoms in the adult. These 'Utah Criteria' are as follows:

I. Childhood Characteristics

A childhood history consistent with ADHD is established through the methods discussed above.

The 'Utah Criteria' require that a patient must have met either the 'narrow' or the 'broad' criteria as a child measured by either the PRS and/or the WURS. The following are those necessary standards for ADD in childhood.

A. Narrow Criteria (DSM-IV)
That the individual meet full DSM-IV criteria for ADHD in childhood.

B. Broad Criteria
Both characteristics 1 and 2, and at least one characteristic from 3 through 6 below:

1 Hyperactivity: more active than other children, unable to sit still, fidgetiness, restlessness, always on the go, talking excessively
2 Attention deficits: sometimes described as a 'short attention span,' distractibility, unable to finish schoolwork
3 Behavior problems in school
4 Impulsivity
5 Overexcitability
6 Temper outbursts

II. Adult Characteristics

The Utah scheme requires that ADHD patients have both symptoms A and B below, plus two of the remaining symptoms (e.g., must be ADHD/Combined Type). At the time of the development of these criteria, Inattentive and the Hyperactive-Impulsive subtypes were not well validated (see above and below). Even now, more work needs to be completed to validate the existence of exclusively Inattentive or Hyperactive-Impulsive subtypes in adults. The reader should also be aware that the Utah criteria are not based exclusively on the behavioral criteria outlined in the DSM because ADHD is viewed as a polythetic condition, consisting of several diverse, non-overlapping features. Thus the criteria also include associated features and subjective symptoms (e.g., low frustration tolerance, temper outbursts, etc.) which the adult undergoing evaluation and his/her partner report [13, 14]. Exactly which symptoms were chosen for inclusion was based upon the best judgment of the senior author. Likewise, the 'cutting point' where a difficulty becomes a symptom was similarly decided. Since this is a reflection of the probable polythetic nature of adult ADHD, it will only become clarified through experience and research which attempts to define a 'pure culture' or 'gold standard' picture of adult ADHD.

A. Motor Hyperactivity
Manifested by restlessness, inability to relax; 'nervousness' (meaning inability to settle down, not anticipatory anxiety); inability to persist in sedentary activities (e.g., watching movies or TV, reading the newspaper); always on the go, dysphoric when inactive.

B. Attention Deficits
Manifested by an inability to keep one's mind on conversations; by distractibility (incapacity to filter extraneous stimuli); difficulty keeping one's mind on reading materials or tasks ('mind frequently somewhere else'); frequent 'forgetfulness'; by often losing or misplacing things; forgetting appointments, plans, car keys, purse, etc.

C. Affective Lability
Usually described as antedating adolescence, and in some instances as far back as the patient can remember. Manifested by definite shifts from a normal mood to depression or mild euphoria or – more often – excitement; depression described as being 'down,' 'bored,' or 'discontented'; anhedonia not present; mood shifts usually last hours to at most a few days and are present without significant physiological concomitants; mood shifts may occur spontaneously or be reactive.

D. Hot Temper, Explosive Short-Lived Outbursts
A hot temper, 'short fuse,' 'low boiling point'; outburst usually followed by quickly calming down. Subjects report that they may have transient loss of control and be

frightened by their own behavior; easily provoked or constant irritability; temper problems interfere with personal relationships.

E. Emotional Overreactivity
Subjects cannot take ordinary stresses in stride and react excessively or inappropriately with depression, confusion, uncertainty, anxiety, or anger; emotional responses interfere with appropriate problem-solving – they experience repeated crises in dealing with routine life stresses; describe themselves as easily 'hassled' or 'stressed out'.

F. Disorganization, Inability to Complete Tasks
A lack of organization and performing on the job, running a household, or performing school work; tasks are frequently not completed; the subject goes from one task to another in haphazard fashion; disorganization in activities, problem-solving, organizing time; lack of 'stick-to-itiveness'.

G. Impulsivity
Minor manifestations include talking before thinking things through; interrupting others' conversations; impatience (e.g., while driving); impulse buying. Major manifestations may be similar to those seen in mania and Antisocial Personality Disorder and include poor occupational performance; abrupt initiation or termination of relationships (e.g., multiple marriages, separations, divorces); excessive involvement in pleasurable activities without recognizing risks of painful consequences (e.g., buying sprees, foolish business investments, reckless driving); inability to delay acting without experiencing discomfort. Subjects make decisions quickly and easily without reflection, often on the basis of insufficient information, to his/her own disadvantage.

H. Associated Features
Associated features include marital instability, academic and vocational success less than expected on the basis of intelligence and education, alcohol and drug abuse, and family histories of ADHD in childhood and parents with alcoholism and Antisocial Personality Disorder.

The Utah Criteria have been chosen to be highly restrictive. Even though we do recognize that ADHD occurs with other psychiatric illnesses, its diagnosis in an adult is only made when other psychological and psychiatric disorders, such as rapid cycling bipolar illness, schizophrenia, etc. have been eliminated. For example, bipolar disorder may coexist with or be mistaken for ADHD. The senior author has treated ADHD patients with Major Depressive Disorder and Bipolar I and II Disorders, yet patients with such comorbid conditions were not included in the development of the Utah Criteria. This stringency in terms of the avoidance of other psychiatric diagnoses is somewhat unique among diagnostic schemas.

Often considered the most stringent of diagnostic schema, the Utah Criteria make childhood hyperactivity continuing into adulthood a mandatory diagnostic symptom.

This criterion obviously eliminates that subgroup of ADHD children and ADHD adults who were, and are, characterized by inattentiveness without hyperactivity and impulsivity. As these criteria were developed prior to the more recent onset of ADHD subtyping, the current Predominantly Inattentive subtype might not fit as well into this framework. For example, the much less stringent criteria used in the rating scale by Biederman relies upon the 18 DSM-IV signs and thus admits a much larger group of patients into research studies. The more stringent requirements were employed in the senior author's research in order to limit investigations to the most clear-cut subgroup of adult patients with ADHD. What was useful, however, for research purposes need not be helpful clinically, because it is clearly the case that many children and adults with inattention alone respond to the same treatments. This also implies a common or related underlying pathophysiology.

A formal diagnosis of adult ADHD using the Utah Criteria is made using the Wender-Reimherr Adult Attention Deficit Disorder Scale (WRAADDS), a structured interview which evaluates the seven symptoms of the Utah Criteria (see appendix C). These symptoms are rated from 0 – not present, 1 – slight, 2 – moderate, 3 – quite a bit, to 4 – very much. A diagnosis of adult ADHD is made if the patient has a rating of 3 or greater on attentional difficulties and hyperactivity and a total score ≥17.

The Utah diagnostic criteria are similarly stringent in excluding patients with certain comorbid psychiatric diagnoses such as Schizophrenia, Antisocial Personality Disorder, and Schizotypal or Borderline Personality Disorders. Again, it was not the intention to thereby deny the frequent comorbidity between ADHD and those conditions [see Klein and Mannuzza, chapter 7]. This rather represented the desire to investigate a more homogeneous sample. Individuals diagnosed with these excluded categories often also have prominent ADHD symptoms and, thus, ADHD remains to be studied in conjunction with such comorbid conditions. Moreover, an important additional area for further investigation is the influence of drug treatment on the ADHD symptoms of adults with comorbid disorders.

Other Common Comorbidities

ADHD children are often comorbid for Conduct Disorder (CD) and most CD children have ADHD as well. While there are many ADHD children without CD, such an elevated association should come as no surprise. This observation is also an important prognostic sign as about one-half of children with CD go on to develop an Antisocial Personality Disorder (APD). Moreover, there appears to be a dose association between ADHD in children and Oppositional Defiant Disorder (ODD), a relationship which may extend into adulthood. Little is known about the value of drug treatment of ADHD in the presence of CD, APD, or ODD, despite reports of the high prevalence of ADHD and some treated ADHD in the criminal population. However, ADHD in children comorbid with CD/ODD appears to respond well to stimulants

[15]. The relationship of adult ADHD with ODD and/or APD requires study [also see Rösler, chapter 8].

Lastly, the Utah studies encountered a high frequency of learning disorders (LD) in the adult ADHD patients. Similar to conduct problems, the continuation of these disorders could have been anticipated because ADHD children have an increased incidence of LDs in reading, spelling, and mathematics as well as expressive language disorders. These skills are rarely assessed in conventional psychiatric evaluations of adults and the degree to which they extend into adulthood remains to be determined. Thus it is often important to evaluate them in adults with ADHD, and to treat them appropriately, since learning disorders often still impact adult life.

It remains an open question as to where to draw the line between which conditions are comorbid with ADHD and which are developmental extensions of this condition. It could well be that some of the presumably independent conditions such as LD and CD which are found in APD represent genetic pleiotropism (a single gene produces multiple effects) and that ADHD as it finally expresses itself is much more polythetic (possessing many features) than previously believed. Just as a single agent, group A streptococci, can produce rheumatic fever that can be expressed through a variety of symptoms such as polyarthritis, Sydenham chorea, myocarditis, endocarditis, and damaged heart valves, so it possible that ADHD may result not only in the symptoms typically associated with it but also 'polythetically' in conditions such as LD and CD. Thus, perhaps the best way to determine the complete signs and symptoms of adult ADHD would be to due longitudinal, follow-up studies. This is a topic very much in need of further research.

Differential Diagnosis

One major diagnostic dilemma will be discussed here: the differentiation between ADHD and other psychiatric diagnoses with very similar symptoms. As indicated previously, differential diagnosis of this disorder is greatly aided by the presence of an 'other' such as spouse, partner, adult children, or parents of the adult patients. Without their observations critical symptoms may be underestimated or simply not disclosed.

Adult ADHD individuals often exhibit depression, affective lability, and irritability. Consequently, ADHD may sometimes be confused with mood disorders such as Bipolar Disorder, Cyclothymic Disorder, and Borderline Personality Disorder (BPD). However, the hypomanic mood shifts typically seen in Cyclothymic Disorder are of weeks or months duration, and differ from the hour-to-hour or day-to-day shifts seen in ADHD. Likewise, anhedonia and physiological concomitants of depression are absent in ADHD, as are the depressive personality traits which Akiskal [16] describes as 'subaffective dysthymia'. Patients with ADHD and BPD appear to share symptoms of impulsivity, affective instability, angry outbursts, and feelings of boredom.

However, both quantitative and qualitative differences are seen between the two diagnostic groups. The impulsivity in ADHD is typically short-lived and thoughtless, rather than 'driven'. Similarly, the ADHD patients' anger is short-lived and episodic, as opposed to the brooding anger typical of the BPD patient. Other major differences between ADHD and BPD patients is that the former do not have the intense conflicted relationships, suicidal preoccupations, self-mutilation, identity disturbances, or feelings of abandonment seen in BPD. Nevertheless, these differences are not clear-cut in all instances, and medications useful in the treatment of ADHD might be of value in treating ADHD-like symptoms in some BPD patients.

A peculiar situation occurs when the patient shares ADHD and Bipolar Disorder (BP). It is increasingly recognized that BP may have its onset in childhood and that a very large fraction of early onset patients with BP have ADHD as well. The import of this is that the ADHD symptoms do not respond to either the mood stabilizers or second generation antipsychotics used for BP. It has been the senior author's experience with several adults with BP whose symptoms have been controlled with medication that they continue to manifest symptoms of ADHD. Cautious addition of stimulants has controlled their ADHD symptoms without exacerbating their BP. This is important because one quarter of adults with BP had childhood BP and most of those also had childhood ADHD. Consider a controlled trial of stimulants if an adult BP patient's symptoms are not well controlled with mood stabilizers and the symptoms that remain have the appearance of ADHD.

Prevalence

There are no definitive epidemiological studies of the prevalence of ADHD in adults. We can, however, reach an order of magnitude calculation for its prevalence from studies estimating the prevalence of ADHD in children and the proportion of these cases that persist into adulthood. Depending on the methodology employed, and the cutoff scores chosen, the prevalence of ADHD in childhood ranges from 3 to 10%. In all studies the disorder is found to be at least 2–3 times as common in boys as in girls. Prevalence rate in different studies varies depending on the setting, the reporter (parent, teacher or self) and the requirements for diagnosis. For example, the prevalence rate is lower when the disorder is required to be pervasive (evident in more than one setting) [17, 18]. Unfortunately, the absence of a diagnostic gold standard limits the determination of the 'true' prevalence of ADHD. That is, we lack the sort of microbiological, pathological, and physiological markers which are often associated with other illnesses, and which permit us to more definitively ascertain the reliability of our diagnosis. It is difficult to meaningfully determine the sensitivity and specificity of our inclusion criteria for ADHD without a means by which to determine whether or not an individual patient 'really' has the disorder. When such a standard is absent, we must make a decision to employ either looser or more stringent criteria. This decision is of course important in terms of determination of prevalence, as well as for determination of which patients we diagnose and subsequently treat. (This question will be further considered in the context of the 'pay-off matrix' in our discussion of treatment.)

The natural history of ADHD as a developmental disorder is best assessed by longitudinal studies of children followed into adult life. There are two relevant studies. Weiss and Hechtman [19] provided adult follow-up at age 25 of 60% of the 'hyperactive' children they had treated when 6–12 years old. Two-thirds of their subjects complained of at least one symptom of restlessness, distractibility, or impulsivity, versus 7% in the controls. Approximately one-half of the patients continued to have moderate or severe problems, while approximately one-quarter had developed Antisocial Personality Disorder. Mannuzza and Klein [13, 20, 21] also followed a cohort of 'hyperactive' children from childhood to ages 18 and 26, and were able to obtain follow-up data from nearly 100%. At age 18, 40% of the patients had ADHD (compared to 3% of the controls), 27% had Conduct Disorder or Antisocial Personality Disorder (versus 8% of the controls), and 16% had non-alcohol Substance Abuse Disorder (vs. 3% of the controls) [22]. By contrast, at age 26 only 11% continued to have full or partial ADHD symptoms, while 18% had Antisocial Personality Disorder, and the same number (16%) continued to have non-alcohol Substance Abuse Disorder [23]. The apparent discrepant results between these two studies [see Klein and Mannuzza, chapter 7] may reflect differences in ADHD severity and/or comorbidity in the groups studied (Klein vs. Weiss). The most striking feature of these studies is the relative persistence of ADHD through adolescence and its apparent decrease in early adult life. This reported drop in the prevalence of ADHD between the ages of 18 and 26 may be interpreted in two different ways. One obvious answer is that the children simply outgrew the disorder. Alternatively this drop may reflect reporter differences, since the investigators depended solely on self-report (of their 25-year-old subjects) for the adult cohort, whereas for child cohorts both the subject and parents were used as informants. In this regard, the Utah studies have consistently found that many adults with persistent ADHD do not report their symptoms or fail to report their severity [24]. From a practical standpoint, the patient's spouses or other informants are also often helpful for initial assessment and in determining treatment response. As the above adult outcome studies were based only on reports from the patients themselves, results likely may have underestimated the true persistence of ADHD in adulthood.

Taken together, the existing prevalence and natural history data suggest that one- to two-thirds of the 3–10% of the childhood prevalence, or somewhere between 1 and 6% of the general population continue to manifest appreciable ADHD symptoms into adult life. It should also be pointed out that these longitudinal studies were begun at a time when the diagnostic criteria of 'hyperactivity' were more narrowly defined. The male subjects so diagnosed might not be representative of more current clinical cohorts which include the 'inattentive subtype', and which may also include more girls and women. No adequate prevalence data are available for these later subjects.

Thus the generalizability of the anterospective studies discussed above, regarding both adult prevalence and prognosis, may be primarily limited to only a subset of the ADHD population.

Presumed Etiology

Genetics

In the early 1970s the senior author advanced the hypothesis that the etiology of 'minimal brain dysfunction' (as ADHD was then often still named) might be genetic in origin and produced by decreased functioning in the catecholaminergic system [25, 26]. Conjectures about a genetic origin were based on an apparently increased frequency of MBD symptoms among the siblings of children with that disorder, as well as an increased frequency of other forms of psychopathology (including alcohol abuse and Antisocial Personality Disorder) among the parents of these patients. In addition, the absence of such psychopathology in the adoptive parents of MBD children suggested the transmission to be genetic in origin.

Since that time there have been many familial studies of ADHD, which allow one to come closer to the relative contributions of genetic versus environment and child-rearing factors. Investigators have looked at the familial association of ADHD; psychopathology in the first-degree relatives of ADHD children; concordance rates between monozygotic and dizygotic twins, and symptoms in foster or adopted children with ADHD. The initial family studies reported an increased frequency of alcohol abuse and Antisocial Personality Disorder among male first-degree relatives and, possibly Somatization Disorder among female biological parents of 'hyperactive' children as compared to controls; as well as an increased frequency of 'hyperactivity' in the siblings of hyperactive children [27–32].

The clustering of ADHD, Antisocial Personality Disorder and alcohol abuse is of interest because family studies conducted by investigators at Washington University found these three disorders to coexist in families, suggesting that the cluster has a genetic basis [33]. Subsequent family studies of ADHD have reported psychopathology in the parents of ADHD children who are comorbid for CD, as well as in the parents of children with 'pure' ADHD. Using other methods, a relationship between ADHD and alcohol abuse was reported by Tarter et al. [34] and Wood et al. [35], both of whom found ADHD to be associated with early-onset alcoholism. Furthermore, Goodman and Stevenson [36] found that the adopted-away sons of alcoholics who were alcoholic were more likely than the non-alcoholics to have had symptoms of 'hyperactivity' in childhood [also see Freitag and Retz, chapter 2]. Finally, a series of recent reports have associated ADHD with an increased family incidence of major affective disorder [37], bipolar disorder [38], conduct disorder [39], and anxiety disorder [40].

Since the familial clustering of psychiatric disorders may be due either to genetic or to environmental influences, other methods are necessary to differentiate between these two modes of transmission. The study of concordance rates for ADHD among monozygotic and dizygotic twins is an effective tool for such investigation. Presumably, since both types of twins share the same familial psychological environment, an increased concordance in the monozygotic pairs (who share a greater degree of genetic material than dizygotic pairs) is due to genetic factors. In a large sample of twins Goodman and Stevenson [36, 41] found an increased concordance of ADHD among monozygotic as compared to dizygotic twins, with an estimate of heritability expressed by genetic linkage to be 64%. More recently, heritability estimates of 75–91% for ADHD, and 60–80% for attention problems on the Child Behavior Checklist have been reported, along with monozygotic concordance rates of 58–83% (versus dizygotic rates of 31 and 47%) [42–44]. These data support transmission of ADHD to be strongly genetic in nature. Monozygotic twins, however, may in fact experience a different psychological environment from that of dizygotic twins, and the twin methodology cannot completely control for this effect. An appropriate strategy to resolve this question is to study foster and adopted children.

Safer [45] investigated the status of full and half-siblings of ADHD children who had been placed in foster care. He found an increase of ADHD-like psychopathology among the siblings which was twice as great among the full as opposed to the half-siblings (as would be expected on genetic grounds). Two other older adoption studies investigated the psychiatric status of the biological parents of children with ADHD, the adoptive parents of children with ADHD, and the biological parents of children without psychiatric disorder [46, 47]. They again found an increased frequency of ADHD-like psychopathology only among the biological parents of ADHD children, while the adoptive parents did not differ from the controls.

The study of adult ADHD by molecular genetic techniques is still in early development and has all been done on children. The genetic interplay in ADHD is complex with over one-half dozen promising candidate genes. Two of the genes currently felt to play a role in adult ADHD is the dopamine receptor D4 gene (DRD4) on chromosome 11 and the dopamine transporter gene (DAT1) on chromosome 5. Although these two genes are perhaps the ones most thoroughly studied as associated with ADHD, they still have a rather low lod score. This may well be due to the high degree of genetic heterogeneity in adult ADHD. Still, even though the lod score is low and even though the probable mechanisms of the genes have not yet been clarified, molecular genetic studies are providing suggestive, but only suggestive [48], evidence of the importance of genes in the etiology and phenomenology of adult ADHD [49].

Taken together, these studies demonstrate the clear presence of genetic factors in the transmission of ADHD and suggest that children with ADHD may be at an increased risk for Antisocial Personality Disorder and alcohol abuse (for more details, see Wender [2]). It should also be noted that ADHD type symptoms can sometimes be caused by other acquired medical conditions such as traumatic brain injury and prenatal or perinatal insult. The biggest potential failing in both making the diagnosis of adult ADHD and then secondarily assessing the condition for a genetic basis is, as with most other psychiatric conditions, the lack of a 'gold standard'; at this point there is no way to know for certain that each of the patients being studied has the same condition, ADHD. This is the problem of any very heterogenous condition and the problem that the Utah Criteria seeks to address.

Catecholamine Hypothesis

Conjectures about the neurophysiological nature of ADHD, or the 'catecholaminergic hypothesis' (see Wender [25] who hypothesized that ADHD with minimal brain dysfunction was a genetically transmitted disorder mediated by decreased catecholaminergic functioning), were based on several observations: the first being reports of the behavioral problems among children who had contracted von Economo's encephalitis during the epidemic of the late teens and early 1920s. Many children who recovered from the acute illness developed a Post-Encephalitic Behavior Disorder with symptoms very similar to those of mixed ADHD and Conduct Disorder. Moreover, adults who recovered from the acute encephalitis frequently displayed symptoms of Parkinson's Disorder. Post-mortem examination of both adults and children who had died from the disorder revealed lesions in the basal ganglia and substantia nigra. These same subcortical brain regions were later linked to idiopathic Parkinson's disorder, which is associated with decreased dopaminergic functioning due to degeneration of dopaminergic neurons.

A second rationale for a dopaminergic hypothesis was the observation that many of the drugs that are most effective in reducing or dramatically eliminating the symptoms of ADHD, the amphetamines and methylphenidate, increase intersynaptic dopamine. As described below, the Utah studies of ADHD adults permitted the investigation of these factors without the risk of exposing children to invasive procedures. One of the first of these studies examined the level of homovanillic acid (HVA), the principal metabolite of dopamine, in the cerebral spinal fluid of adults with ADHD and in controls [50]. As was also the case for people with Parkinson's disorder, decreased levels of HVA were found in ADHD adults who had responded to treatment with methylphenidate. By contrast, increased levels of HVA were found in the non-responding ADHD patients. This replicated the results of two earlier smaller studies in 'hyperactive' children and in children with minimal brain dysfunction [51, 52].

The second approach was to administer drugs with a comparatively specific action in patients with ADHD. The hypothesized relevant neurotransmitter dopamine is metabolized in the brain by monoamine oxidase B (MAO-A metabolizes serotonin, norepinephrine, and dopamine). In relatively low to moderate doses, two MAO inhibitors – pargyline (no longer marketed) and L-deprenyl (selegiline) – are specific MAO-B inhibitors, although in high doses they may affect MAO-A as well. Correspondingly, it was found that in low doses both drugs produced moderate-to-marked improvement in about 60% of ADHD adults [35, 55]. Since at low levels these drugs presumably increase the availability of dopamine and do not increase levels of serotonin and norepinephrine, the results also support the dopaminergic hypothesis.

Further trials of selegiline (now available as an orphan drug but available in a patch) may be of interest although the likelihood of its utility seems limited.

Treatment

Medication

The Utah group has conducted placebo-controlled and open-label drug trials in over 300 patients, including over 225 ADHD patients treated with stimulants. These include four double-blind placebo-controlled trials: three of methylphenidate with varying subject numbers and one of 48 patients with pemoline [2, 24, 56, 57]. In addition, the Utah group treated 79 patients in open-label trials: pargyline, L-deprenyl (selegiline), bupropion, levodopa, D,L-phenylalanine, and L-tyrosine [35, 53–55, 58, 59].

In crossover design studies about 60–70% of patients receiving stimulant medication showed moderate-to-marked improvement, as compared with 20% of those receiving placebo. These degrees of responsivity were reflected in Global Assessment of Functioning (GAF) scores in patients with moderate-to-marked improvement. The average pre-treatment GAF scores in the studies are about 55 (moderate symptoms) and post-treatment scores were about 75 (slight symptoms present only in reaction to stress). As mentioned, open studies of pargyline and selegiline in 27 patients found, again, that about 60% exhibited moderate-to-marked improvement to treatment with an MAO inhibitor. Lastly, a therapeutic trial of bupropion in 19 patients, who had previously responded to stimulants or MAO inhibitors, found that approximately half responded to bupropion and decided to remain on that drug [60]. More recently, Wilens et al. repeated these results with bupropion [61] and long-acting bupropion XL [62].

Turning to less dopaminergic drugs, the tricyclic antidepressants have generally not been useful in adults (or children). Children displayed an immediate response, but after 6–8 weeks became tolerant to the drug despite increased dose. Adults also seemed less tolerant of the side effects of these drugs than are depressed patients; complaining of the anticholinergic effects, weight gain, and impaired sexual functioning. Thus, they may be more effective than placebo but the magnitude of change is low compared to stimulants. SSRIs appear to be of no value in ADHD patients who are not depressed or dysthymic, but may be of considerable benefit for those with comorbid depression or dysthymia. Atomoxetine and modafinil have shown some early success in treating ADHD children [63, 64] but have only modestly to moderately demonstrated effectiveness in the treatment of ADHD adults when compared to stimulants.

There have been three attempts to replicate the Utah treatment studies. Mattes et al. [65] conducted a placebo-controlled trial of methylphenidate in 66 patients, but did not demonstrate a favorable response to the drug. There are several reasons why this may have occurred. Sampling variables may be a factor: 60% of the sample did not meet the criteria of childhood 'hyperactivity' employed in the Utah studies and thus may have met diagnoses other than ADHD. Moreover, many of the patients were comorbid for substance abuse and BPD, patients who would have been excluded in the Utah studies. More recently, Spencer et al. [66, 67] were able to replicate the Utah findings with methylphenidate in a placebo-controlled trial of 146 subjects, and Rösler et al. [68] could demonstrate robust treatment effects of methylphenidate over 24 weeks in another placebo-controlled trial.

Taken together, these studies clearly demonstrate the efficacy of methylphenidate, dextroamphetamine, and possibly selegiline (it is now available and likely to be used) in the treatment of adults with ADHD. However, although several medications have shown some effectiveness in treating adult ADHD, the stimulants are unquestionably the most effective and the drugs of choice. Both dextroamphetamine and methylphenidate in one of its many formulations may be very effective but either one may not be effective in a particular patient. If one fails, in most cases the next step is to try the other stimulant. This should be done routinely since which stimulant is likely to be useful is unpredictable.

After evaluation and a discussion of the patient's level of symptoms, the senior author utilizes the therapeutic pay-off matrix alluded to previously, i.e., the benefits and liabilities of a therapeutic trial of medication when he does or does not have the disorder. A consideration of the four possibilities reveals that the risks of treating a patient who does not have ADHD are minimal, while there are considerable disadvantages to not offering a trial of treatment to someone with the disorder. The above holds with the proviso that the use of stimulant drugs does not lead to abuse of those medications (fortunately, ADHD patients do not get 'high' with stimulants; an additional diagnostic feature of ADHD). For this reason, stimulants should be used cautiously or not at all in persons with a history of drug abuse. In general, however, it is emphasized that therapeutic trials are warranted whenever the diagnosis seems probable because the benefits can be assessed rapidly. Equally important, given the numerous conditions comorbid with ADHD, further research must be done on medication in the treatment of ADHD associated with these related conditions.

The Utah group has used a structured interview to assess adult ADHD symptoms and their changes in our treatment studies [2]. Symptom changes seen with effective treatment include the following:

1 *Hyperactivity* – Fidgeting and restlessness decrease; patients are able to relax; then are able to stay at their desks or at the dinner table or in a movie or in church.
2 *Inattention* – Concentration is greatly improved. It is not only that patients can concentrate better; they can concentrate when they want to. Distractibility diminishes or disappears. Attention to spousal conversation improves and frequently is quickly manifested in better marital relations.
3 *Mood lability* – Both highs and lows decrease, as do feelings of boredom; mood is described as 'level' or 'stable.'

4 *Temper* – The threshold for outbursts is raised. Patients are less irascible and their angry outbursts are less frequent, less extreme, and frequently disappear altogether.
5 *Disorganization* – Organizational activities improve. This is evident at school, in running a household, in vocational function. Patients may spontaneously establish orderly strategies.
6 *Stress sensitivity* – Patient's self-descriptions include having their thin skin thickened, able to take life problems in their stride, feeling less 'hassled' about daily existence.
7 *Impulsivity* – Patients report that they do not interrupt others while listening to them (another feature that improves conversations and relationships), that they think before they speak, that they have become tolerant drivers and that they stop impulse buying.

Practically speaking, ADHD is a life-long disorder and the duration of drug treatment may also be life-long [69]. Amphetamines have been used since 1937 with no long-term toxicities reported. However, both methylphenidate and D-amphetamine increase heart rate and blood pressure, which must be carefully monitored in adult patients. Their use may require adjuvant therapy to control heart rate and blood pressure. Whether such drugs interfere with the therapeutic action of the stimulants remains to be demonstrated.

Psychosocial Interventions

Appropriate management of adult patients with ADHD involves more than adequate drug therapy alone. Similar to the case for children, the best treatment involves education about the disorder and psychotherapy addressing concomitant problems. Once the diagnosis has been made, we help patients recognize how ADHD is manifested in their current behavior. As the therapeutic relationship develops, discussion may broadened to include the role played by ADHD characteristics in the patient's life history, including academic and vocational choices, friendships, sexual relationships, and functioning as a spouse and as a parent. ADHD symptomatology may be intimately woven into all these aspects of life, and it takes patients much time – during continuing treatment – to identify and understand its contributions to their life story.

In educating patients we also help them understand that the chronic nature of the disorder has likely resulted in their developing compensatory techniques which are no longer adaptive. These maladaptive techniques may resolve spontaneously with pharmacotherapy, or they may require psychotherapeutic intervention. Supportive problem-directed therapy, behavioral intervention, coaching, or cognitive remediation can help with these problems [see Richter et al., chapter 9]. Couple therapy and/or family therapy may be useful. Finally, ADHD does not prevent one from having other psychological problems and these may be more apparent, or therapeutically accessible, after the symptoms of ADHD have remitted with medication. In short, concurrent supportive psychosocial treatment can be key.

Case histories of successful diagnosis and treatment are easy to come by these days. Below are two examples of such successes; one in a young woman and a second in an elderly man with comments by his wife. Recognize that treatment of ADHD with stimulants can produce some of the most dramatic positive effects in psychiatry.

Case Histories

Case I

A young woman was 18 years old when, prompted by her social worker aunt, she contacted our adult ADHD clinic. Her young life had already been seriously disrupted. She had abused alcohol and marijuana between the ages of 12 and 16. Although she had superior intelligence, she had dropped out of high school (secondary school) after 2 years. At the ages of 15 and 17 she had two out of wedlock pregnancies. Her mother had thrown her out of the house and currently she was eking out an existence on welfare. She entered a double-blind placebo crossover trial of methylphenidate and placebo and showed no improvement on placebo, then was 'very much' improved on methylphenidate. She was maintained to her substantial benefit on methylphenidate with the following changes in her life.

She decided that she had made a serious mistake in dropping out of school and applied for and acquired a general equivalency diploma (GED; formal testing equivalent to that required for secondary school graduation). When she expressed the desire to work, her mother forgave her and the patient came home where her mother could help take care of the 2 children. The patient began in an office (she did have secretarial skills) and after 2 years was promoted to a higher position. At this juncture, she was the beneficiary of great luck. (Luck plays an essential role in human affairs but is never discussed as an important determinant of one's fate by psychiatrists.) She met a young computer engineer who wanted to marry her – despite assuming responsibility of the 2 stepchildren – and shortly thereafter she expressed a wish to attend college. She easily passed the entrance requirements at the university and after 4 years was graduated with such high marks that she was given a tuition grant to attend graduate school in cognitive psychology. Two years ago, she contacted me to tell me that she had received a second grant. Her marriage was going smoothly, her children were adjusting well to their less disordered life and she was very happy.

Case II: George F.

Clinical Background

George F. is 49 years old and had been in the methylphenidate study for 3 years. George is adopted, and his family history is unknown. His symptoms at intake were varied and severe. He loved to read but was unable to do much, owing to attention and concentration difficulties. Professionally he has lost numerous jobs because of failure to complete important projects on time, and restlessness and fidgetiness that caused him to (literally) jump around. Extreme disorganization at work and at home were major chronic problems; in fact, he and his wife have separate bedrooms because she can't stand his messiness. His wife describes him as chronically irritable, hyperreactive to sounds that don't bother most people and periodically explosive at home and at work. 'The kids never know when or at what he's going to explode'.

Emotionally he was mildly depressed, expressed feelings of guilt and inadequacy about letting his family down, but seemed *not to worry* about problems his wife felt he should be worrying about. She was particularly upset about his pattern of making impulsive, inappropriate remarks in social settings that his few close friends put up with and that he didn't understand were inappropriate until much later, if at all. These severe difficulties continued to plague George even after 7 years of psychotherapy.

He has been receiving 40 mg of methylphenidate per day (10 mg every 3 h, 4 times per day), and after 3 years in our study showed these changes: his score on the Global Assessment of Functioning has risen from 56 to 80, and his score on the Social Adjustment Scale has improved from moderate maladjustment [4] to good [2].

Statement of George F.

The controversy surrounding Attention Deficit Disorder is certainly understandable. Those who haven't experienced it personally or through their children are only aware of the various issues through the simplified media coverage. I know. Even though I have the disorder, it took me a long time to realize that my various struggles could be much more than mere lack of self-discipline. From my understanding of the disorder through the press, I initially felt I didn't suffer from ADD since I didn't manifest the most obvious symptom: hyperactivity. After all, the other symptoms seem common to everyone to some degree or some of the time. It is hard for most people to comprehend that for a few of us these symptoms are constant and debilitating. It is not a simple disease like the measles or the common cold. We who suffer are so used to the struggle that we are unaware that we are not functioning at a level that others take for granted.

Like most critics, I thought that ADD was just another fashionable trend in medicine. I felt that taking a magic pill that could change the way your mind works was naïve. It was the easy answer for those who were merely avoiding the hard work of learning the skills of concentration, developing good work habits, and simply taking responsibility for one's immaturity. I distrusted drugs in general. Unlike most of my friends in the 60s, I didn't take marijuana or LSD. I didn't want to give up what little control I had over my behavior.

For most of my life I held onto the belief that I could change my poor work habits if I could just find the right method of self-discipline. When I began to realize that all the efforts I had made to try to become more efficient, more focused, and more attentive were not working, I reached the level of profound despair. Nothing worked. To make things worse, my wife shared that despair. My marriage and family life were on the verge of failure, and I lost all hope.

Like many adult sufferers of ADD, it took outside pressure from my spouse to force me to submit to diagnostic tests. Even after I was accepted into the University of Utah's ADD study group, I had lingering doubts about its worth. I was relieved to have a medical explanation for what I had considered serious personality flaws. However, a lifetime of dashed hopes had left me skeptical about much benefit from a mere pill. I took part in a double-blind test for 4 months. Neither the doctor nor I knew if I was taking placebos or Ritalin.

The first 2 months were discouraging, since I figured that at least one of the monthly supply of pills must of been Ritalin. There was no discernible difference in my behavior in either month. I received the third bottle of pills in November of 1992. Without much confidence, I took the first pill of this group that evening before I relaxed in my bedroom to read a difficult book that had stymied me for over a month. I didn't feel anything at all from the pill. Somehow I expected a palpable rise in my awareness, a change in my mood or a bit of a high since Ritalin is, after all, a stimulant. So, I forgot about the pill, dismissing it again as worthless. Soon my wife called me to dinner, a little earlier than usual, I thought. I looked at my watch and realized nearly an hour had passed. As I marked my place in the book, I noticed with shock that I had read 30 pages without once losing my train of thought. This may not seem significant to most avid readers but to me it was astonishing. Although I read a great deal, it has always been a struggle for me. Only truly good fiction holds my attention for more than a paragraph. But I had read this particularly turgid non-fiction at a much faster rate than I had ever read any of my favorite books.

I became a believer in the miracle drug Ritalin. Why don't people accept such a possibility when we all know that other drugs are equally amazing? We take aspirin for granted as one of the most effective medicines for pain, but no one has been able to discover how it works. This cheap, simple drug is now being recognized as helpful in controlling heart disease and preventing strokes.

During that next month other subtle changes occurred that were much more apparent to my wife and children. Before I describe the many ways this drug has affected my life, I have to give you an idea what my struggles were like for the previous four decades.

The first clear memory I have of my lack of attention was in fifth grade. I know it was obvious earlier because my mother told me that even my second grade teacher commented on my 'daydreaming'. But in fifth grade, I remember a specific day when we were reading silently in class about Mexico. As I was reading, I remember feeling anxious that I wouldn't finish the assignment before the class day ended. I kept looking at the clock to see how much time was left and trying to push myself to read faster. I looked at my neighbors' books and noticed that they were much farther ahead than I. There was a wonderful photograph of a lush mountainside with a man taking a loaded donkey down a narrow trail. I began to think about being there on that trail, feeling the hot Mexican sun, and hearing the birds in the trees.

Soon I was thinking about the canyon near my home that cuts into the city from the foothills of the Wasatch Mountains. I remember seeing the Denver-Rio Grande train going past the swimming hole one day of the previous summer. I looked out the window to see if the weather was good enough to go down there that day right after school. My teacher noticed me gazing out the window and asked me if I had finished already. She became angry when I said no and took me out into the hall. She gave me a stern lecture about my lack of 'stick-to-itiveness' and embarrassed me deeply. I remember vowing to never let that happen ever again. But, despite all my efforts, it occurred over and over again, even through college. Every time I caught my mind wandering from the text, I would try to force myself to focus. It never worked. In minutes my mind would be on another track. It was apparent that the harder I tried, the more anxious I became, which inevitably caused me to think about not getting finished and imagining the consequences instead of focusing. It never occurred to me that there was anything I could do besides vowing to learn how to change my bad habits. But none of the study techniques I tried seemed to help. I generally approached my work in a state of panic, spending late hours trying to catch up, and developing a chronic case of diarrhea.

All through school I never finished a single textbook. I specifically recall being desperate about chemistry. Despite my intense determination to do well I was only able to read two of the 17 chapters assigned for that year. I still managed to get a C in the class. In most of my classes, I survived purely by my wits. Fortunately, my memory for facts has been phenomenal and compensated for my inability to focus on my reading. Taking notes was a disaster since it got in the way of my listening. Since I got good grades, my parents never worried about my work and never pushed me to do better. They were just happy that I wasn't a poor student like my three brothers. They didn't suspect that I was having difficulties.

They didn't have to push me because I already did so myself, mercilessly. I would consistently stay up to one or two in the morning to work on assignments which should have taken half the time. I would come to school exhausted, often with my work unfinished. Teachers regularly gave me good grades on my incomplete papers because it was obvious that I understood the assignments. Report cards would usually comment on my incompletes, that I was capable of doing much better.

Because I loved literature, my favorite class was English. I eventually majored in English in college. I often came early to my favorite high school English teacher's class to talk about what we were reading in class and about other fiction as well. Despite my constant lack of full preparation I would still find time to read other things. She told me near the end of the year that I had a wonderful mind for literature but it was too bad that I didn't work hard enough. I remember thinking that I couldn't possibly work any harder.

One symptom I never had to any great degree was hyperactivity. Perhaps if I had, my ADD would have been recognized earlier in life. Of course, in the 1950s and early 1960s, hyperactivity was not yet considered anything more than poor behavior. The most I would do was bounce my leg rapidly in my chair or tap my pencil. This would irritate my parents, and later my wife, but I was only admonished to quit doing it. I could sit at my desk without jumping up and running around like other ADD kids.

However, I was very impulsive. When my mind wandered away from the immediate tasks at hand I would think of other things I needed to do and drop what I was doing and pursue the distracting interest. Too many things had the capacity to distract me from the more crucial tasks. In a perverse way, this was often beneficial to my education. For instance, whenever I read an unfamiliar word, I would immediately look it up in the dictionary. Words have always fascinated me. However, once in the dictionary, I would look up synonyms, antonyms, and the etymologies of the word I was researching. Often the simple goal of looking up a single word would take half an hour or more. Although my vocabulary and spelling skills grew to be impressive, I wouldn't be able to finish reading anything within a reasonable time. Distractions would also benefit my later interest in architecture. The tendency to go off on a different angle would aid my designs because my divergent thinking often lead to unique ideas and other possibilities that could not be predicted in a strictly linear approach. Unfortunately, precious time would be lost, and I would have to work long hours to synthesize these ideas into a coherent whole. Usually this would leave me exhausted and many of the details needed to complete the design would be poorly thought out.

Usually the content of my reading would stimulate related, but diverging thoughts. This helped me to gain better insights about literature through analogy. Mention of an unfamiliar event, topic, or person would drive me to my encyclopedia in another time-consuming digression.

This was also particularly noticeable in my speech. If I were talking with someone about some idea I would often veer off the track in mid-sentence with a related point. This would generally lead to yet another diverging explanation until I would lose all sense of my original direction. While listening to others, I would be thinking of my next thought, which I feared would vanish before I had time to respond. I would blurt out before the speaker had a chance to finish his point.

Since my mother also had this annoying tendency, our conversations were particularly chaotic. She would complain that I didn't have a clutch on my tongue, that my speech would jerk into motion before I engaged my mind. Of course, her habit of finishing my sentences for me while I was searching for the right words drove me crazy.

Needless to say, my social skills did not develop in a normal manner. Many people would gradually drift away from me while I tried to talk to them. I tended to keep quiet whenever I met new people. Parties were never much fun. I was particularly uncomfortable when I met anyone who spoke with grace and ease. By the time I graduated from high school I was so resentful of the popular students that I was becoming bitter, sarcastic and deeply depressed. I not only had not gained any confidence in myself but I began to lose hope that I would ever be able to perform the tasks necessary for success in any field that I wanted to pursue. When teachers or employers would give me instructions, my mind would often be racing along unproductive directions. I would try to take extensive notes during and after instructions but they were inevitably chaotic and difficult to read.

My attempts to organize my work led me to try many different techniques that would have been effective for the average person. But they rarely worked for me. I would be thinking of too many things at the same time and be frustrated about learning how to make priorities. Despite the many files I organized, I would usually lose some crucial bit of information and waste my energy trying to recover it. I became fanatical about having all the information I needed to finish a project. If I didn't know an answer to some matter, its importance would grow into an obsession. I grew more and more unable to make simple decisions.

Despite all my problems I managed to receive a degree in English literature and later a Masters in architecture. After I got my professional license, I began to believe that maybe I had grown out of my bad habits. However, they continued to persist and even got worse. Becoming an adult did not end my ADD. Of course, I didn't realize that my problem had a neurological basis. I continued to feel depressed about the pervasive nature of my problems. Nothing seemed to work for me. In 20 years of professional practice, I did not advance to the level of income, performance, and ability that I knew I was capable of achieving if I could only work productively. I resented my colleagues who did much better than I, those whose design abilities were less than mine. Of course, I rationalized, they knew how to use the system better than I. I became very adept at finding excuses for losing jobs, blaming others for my failures.

I turned this on to my wife as well. My negativity almost destroyed my marriage. I blamed her for being too difficult, too demanding. I realize now how badly I abused her trust and love. Even though I knew she had the right to expect me to be home when I said I would be, my inability to predict how long the project would take drove her to despair. It was so hard to keep my work timely and give her and our children the attention they deserved. My frustration with work left me irritable with my family. Often, I would explode in unpredictable anger. Thankfully, they kept their faith in me long enough for me to discover the possibility that I had ADD.

It would be an exaggeration to claim that my life has changed overnight into a wonderful dream since I have been on Ritalin, but the long nightmare is at last over. Although I still have a lot to relearn about organization, time management, social skills, and obsession with detail, I no longer feel despair or anxiety. I can now make reasonable estimates about the time necessary to complete projects and finish them without resorting to long anxiety-ridden nights. My relationships with my employers and fellow workers have improved significantly. I'm more cooperative and attentive to their needs. Architecture has now become the delightful profession I had long ago wished it would be. I no longer drag myself to work late and exhausted because I stayed up late trying to catch up.

Ritalin literally saved my marriage and my relationships with my children and close friends. I pay attention to them without getting defensive, critical, or insensitive. The last 3 years with my wife have been a marvelous restoration of our initial love for each other. We share much more time with each other and her trust in me continues to grow. I no longer keep her waiting up for me past the time I have told her that I would be home. I don't make us late for movies or parties because I always know where I leave my keys now. She tells me her feelings and without fear that I will criticize them as irrational, which they never were.

Distractions still occur, of course, but I do not impulsively respond to them. I have limited my non-architectural interests to those that are important to me. I have enjoyed researching a particular social problem (not ADD) that I have deeply cared about for 11 years. My writing about it has received recognition from the international press and a growing audience of those intimately involved in it. One of the rewards of this effort has been several opportunities to travel and speak to the public. Last year I went all the way to Melbourne, Australia, to speak to the Victorian Parliament, several other groups, and to the press.

This is amazing to me since I had never been comfortable speaking about ideas for fear that I would make a complete fool of myself. I can confidently speak to many people at once and maintain a coherent direction without confusing them with digressions. This is immensely satisfying after a lifetime of being unable to express myself.

As I said at the start, I can understand the lack of acceptance of ADD as neurological disorder and the effectiveness of its treatment through a mere drug. Unless someone has gone through the agony of my experiences, it is difficult to accept. I can only hope that critics can suspend judgment about this until more evidence is gathered. I am confident that it will be appreciated in the near future and that the medical profession will finally recognized the validity of the diagnosis and its treatment. Scientific revolutions have often been dismissed as false, even blasphemous. Galileo, Darwin, Pasteur, and many others had suffered the outrageous criticism that ADD researchers are now receiving from reactionary groups like the Church of Scientology. For the sake of the thousands of sufferers of Attention Deficit Disorder, both children and adults, I hope that sympathy and understanding will soon prevail over the hysterical forces of ignorance. They deserve the right to experience a life relatively free from confusion and despair.

Comment by Spouse of George F.

It's always been hard to put my finger on exactly what was so difficult about living with George. By all standards, he was the ideal mate; he worked hard, was faithful, wasn't abusive, was highly intelligent and extremely good-looking. My complaints were those of every married woman: he was uncommunicative, he kept me waiting for hours, he didn't care about my feelings, our way of managing money and disciplining children were diametrically opposed, etc.

The problems were run of the mill but abnormal in the sense that they were extreme and unrelenting, e.g. he would estimate that he had 3 or 4 hours of work before coming home but it turned out to be 18 hours, an 'all-nighter.'

My emotional history made me very vulnerable to someone not showing up. I would be in a state of panic for hours. Even though I told George how much I suffered when he kept me waiting, he never changed his behavior.

I could never count on him to be on time, to help me with decisions or with children. He just could not attend to his inner world and to the rest of the problems of living.

One night we came home at midnight and our 13-year-old son was playing catch at the corner. I yelled at him to come home. He didn't. I asked George to deal with the problem and he got furious with me for yelling, thereby disturbing the neighbors.

An angry tone of voice always irritated him. Once he got mad because the sound of my daughter chewing croutons irritated him. It took hours of discussion for me to convince him to be reasonable. I thought that I was the one who was lacking in relating and communicating skills. This eroded my self-esteem. His behavior was unpredictable, impulsive and almost completely unresponsive to outside influence. Raising my voice, confrontation, asserting my needs, explaining, getting angry, moving out twice, not only failed to get my needs met but resulted in his asserting that I was the 'bad guy'.

A typical scenario occurred the summer our 12-year-old daughter was in a recital at a music camp in St. George. After the 5-hour drive, George arrived rather disheveled and his appearance caused our daughter some embarrassment.

The next day we were attending the recital and after examining the program, George assumed that he would have time to go get a haircut before Jennifer's turn. After 16 years of marriage I knew that it was useless to advise him not to do this. So he went and of course missed her performance. After everything was over, he insisted that she go to the piano and play the piece for him so that he could get a picture. She was upset and uncooperative and George was irritated.

As my psychiatrist put it, being around George was like 'having to walk on eggshells.'

The stresses of any change in his routine (like a vacation) exacerbated his condition: Once he lost a contact lens while taking it out at dusk at a windswept roadside stop; another time, he left his wallet on top of the car and lost it, thus ruining our skiing holiday. In France, he got so angry when a driver tailgated and passed us, that he had to follow the driver and do the same thing. He was not a mean person and as long as I left him alone and didn't need anything from him, he was fine and quite mellow. He couldn't tolerate the mildest of stresses of family life. The unremitting nature of his impulsive and irrational behavior and the inability to grow and develop into a fully sharing partner are the factors that made our problems different from the usual marital difficulties.

After 23 years of marriage plus 3 years of courtship, and after George had been in psychoanalysis for 7 years, I was ready to die: I had gotten nowhere in my various careers and I couldn't love the man to whom I had committed so much of my life.

And then one final crisis and the miracle of the ADD diagnosis and the Ritalin cure occurred.

I had left my job when George had managed to hang on to a job for 2 years. Our daughter had been accepted at Yale and then, once again, he was laid off (the 17th time in 18 years).

This time, finally, I came to the certain conclusion that my husband suffered from a neurological problem. It had become imperative that he be correctly diagnosed and somehow taught to adapt to his handicap.

My conversations with George, like everyone else's, were difficult to impossible. Either he said nothing but yes or no to questions that would normally require elaboration, or he would go on and on and on about whatever topic had grabbed his interest at the moment, with no desire for input from the person who was listening to him. If I expressed disinterest even with just a look, he would become defensive.

I concluded that his disorder was very much analogous to being deaf as he seemed to not perceive other human beings' non-verbal language and expectations.

The changes in George's behavior in the two and a half years he's been on Ritalin are as hard to describe as it is to describe the disorder. They are very subtle but the children and I can tell as soon as he opens his mouth whether or not he's taken the medication.

Mainly, he isn't so defensive; he doesn't get his dander up at every little thing that doesn't go his way. He listens, and he shuts up when he perceives that no one wants to listen to him. He is more spontaneous and invites me to share in some of his activities. He is accepting when I decline.

He always worked very hard and was phenomenally energetic. He never seemed to tire. Whereas before he dissipated his energy going from one project to another, focusing on his interest rather than on results, now he completes project after project: gardening, remodeling the house, writing, and of course his professional duties.

In summary, I really can't find the words to express what a difference George's treatment with Ritalin has made in my life. The very first pill was more effective than 26 years of love and patience and understanding and 7 years of psychotherapy.

I have a Masters degree in neurophysiology and have worked for nearly 30 years in neuroscience or as a teacher of disturbed adolescents. I am an expert on Freud. I would never have believed that a drug could have such a profound effect on someone's behavior.

First of all, I thought that a drug's action would be too global to be effective. Secondly, I thought George's problems stemmed from having been brought up in a dysfunctional family and that he needed to learn new behaviors.

Now I am convinced that Ritalin affects the firing of neurons such that perception of the outside world is different than it is without the medication.

I hope these few pages succeed in showing my gratitude to Dr. Wender and his research team.

Conclusion

The take-away message from this overview is that ADHD in adults is a common genetically transmitted neurological disorder, which is probably mediated by decreased brain dopaminergic functioning. It is usually undiagnosed, but it can be diagnosed fairly easily and can resemble or coexist with other psychiatric disorders. At least 60% of patients experience a substantial, and in many instances a dramatic, response to drug treatment, and such drug treatment can make ADHD patients more amenable to a number of psychotherapeutic approaches. The benefits of combined treatment may be of life-changing proportions.

References

1 Wender PH: Attention-deficit hyperactivity disorder in adults. Psychiatr Clin N Am 1998;21:761–774.

2 Wender PH: Attention-Deficit Hyperactivity Disorder in Adults. New York, Oxford University Press, 1995.

3 Still GF: Some abnormal psychical conditions in children. Lancet 1902;E:1008–1012, 1077–1082, 1163–1168.

4 Douglas VI: Stop, look, and listen: the problem of sustained attention and impulse control in hyperactive and normal children. Can J Behav Sci 1972; 4:259–282.

5 American Psychiatric Association (APA): Diagnostic and Statistical Manual of Mental Disorders, ed 3. Washington, APA, 1980.

6 Barkley RA: ADHD adolescents: family conflicts and their treatment. Grant from National Institute of Mental Health, MH41583, 1990.

7 Hynd GW, Lorys AR, Semrund-Chileman M, et al: Attention deficit disorder without hyperactivity: a distinct behavioral and neurocognitive syndrome. J Child Neurol 1991;6:S37–S43.

8 Lahey BB, Carlson CL: Validity of the diagnostic category of attention deficit disorder without hyperactivity: a review of the literature; in Shaywitz SE, Shaywitz BA (eds): Attention Deficit Disorder Comes of Age: Towards the 25th Century. Austin/TX, Pro-Ed, 1992, pp 119–144.

9 American Psychiatric Association (APA): Diagnostic and Statistical Manual of Mental Disorders, ed 4. Washington, APA, 1994.

10 Conners CK: Rating scales; in Psychopharmacology Bulletin: Special Issue on Pharmacotherapy of Children: Washington, NIMH, Government Printing Office, 1973.

11 Ward MF, Wender PH, Reimherr FW: The Wender Utah Rating Scale: an aid in the retrospective diagnosis of attention deficit hyperactivity disorder. Am J Psychiatry 1993;150:885–890.

12 Retz-Junginger P, Retz W, Blocher D, et al: Reliability and validity of the Wender Utah Rating Scale Short Form. Retrospective assessment of symptoms for attention deficit/hyperactivity disorder. Nervenarzt 2003;74:987–993.

13 Mannuzza, S, Klein RG, Konig PH, et al: Hyperactive boys almost grown up. IV. Criminality and its relationship to psychiatric status. Arch Gen Psychiatry 1989;46:1073–1079.

14 Curran S, Fitzgerald M: Attention deficit hyperactivity disorder in the prison population (letter). Am J Psychiatry 1999;156:1664–1665.

15 Jensen PS, Hinshaw SP, Kraemer HC, et al: ADHD comorbidity findings from the MTA study: comparing comorbid subgroups. J Am Acad Child Adolesc Psychiatry 2001;40:147–158.

16 Akiskal HS: Dysthymic disorder: psychopathology of proposed chronic depressive subtypes. Am J Psychiatry 1983;140:11–20.

17 Sherman DK, McGue MK, Iacono WG: Twin concordance for attention deficit hyperactivity disorder: a comparison of teachers' and mothers' reports. Am J Psychiatry 1997;154:532–535.

18 Schachar R, Rutter M, Smith A: The characteristics of situationally and pervasively hyperactive children: implications for syndrome definition. J Child Psychol Psychiatry 1981;22:375–392.

19 Weiss G, Hechtman LT: Hyperactive Children Grown Up: ADHD in Children, Adolescents, and Adults. New York, The Guilford Press, 1993.

20 Mannuzza S, Klein RG, Bessler A, et al: Adult outcome of hyperactive boys: educational achievement, occupational rank, and psychiatric status. Arch Gen Psychiatry 1993;50:565–576.

21 Mannuzza S, Klein RG: Long-term prognosis in attention-deficit/hyperactivity disorder. Child Adolescent Psychiatr Clin N Am 2000;9:711–726.

22 Gittelman R, Mannuzza S, Shenker R, Bonagura N: Hyperactive boys almost grown up. I. Psychiatric status. Arch Gen Psychiatry 1985;42:937–947.

23 Mannuzza S, Klein RG, Bonagura N, et al: Hyperactive boys almost grown up. V. Replication of psychiatric status. Arch Gen Psychiatry 1991;48: 77–83.

24 Wender PH, Reimherr FW, Wood DR: Attention deficit disorder ('minimal brain dysfunction') in adults: a replication study of diagnosis and drug treatment. Arch Gen Psychiatry 1981;38:449–456.

25 Wender PH: Minimal Brain Dysfunction in Children. New York, Wiley, 1971.

26 Wender PH: The minimal brain dysfunction syndrome in children. I. The syndrome and its relevance for psychiatry. II. A psychological and biochemical model for the syndrome. J Nerv Ment Dis 1972;155:55–71.

27 Cantwell DP: Psychiatric illness in the families of hyperactive children. Arch Gen Psychiatry 1972;27: 414–417.

28 Morrison JR, Stewart MA: The psychiatric status of the legal families of adoptive hyperactive children. Arch Gen Psychiatry 1973;28:888–891.

29 Morrison J: Adult psychiatric disorders in parents of hyperactive children and controls. Am J Psychiatry 1980;137:825–827.

30 Biederman J, Faraone SV, Keenan K, et al: Further evidence for family-genetic risk factors in attention deficit hyperactivity disorder. Patterns of comorbidity in probands and relatives in psychiatrically and pediatrically referred samples. Arch Gen Psychiatry 1992;49:728–738.
31 Faraone SV, Biederman J, Chen WJ, et al: Segregation analysis of attention deficit hyperactivity disorder. Psychiatr Genet 1992;2:257–275.
32 Comings D: Clinical and molecular genetics of ADHD & Tourette's syndrome: two related polygenic disorders. Ann NY Acad Sci 2001;93L.
33 Guze SB: Criminality and Psychiatric Disorders. New York, Oxford University Press, 1976.
34 Tarter RE, McBride H, Buonpane N, et al: Differentiation of alcoholics: childhood history of minimal brain dysfunction, family history, and drinking pattern. Arch Gen Psychiatry 1977;34:761–768.
35 Wood DR, Reimherr FW, Wender PH: The use of L-deprenyl in the treatment of attention deficit disorder-residual type (ADD-RT). Psychopharmacol Bull 1983;19:627–629.
36 Goodman R, Stevenson J: A twin study of hyperactivity. I. An examination of hyperactivity scores and categories derived from rider teacher and parent questionnaires. J Child Psychol Psychiatry 1989;30: 671–689.
37 Biederman J, Faraone SV, Keenan K, et al: Evidence of familial association between attention deficit disorder and major affective disorders. Arch Gen Psychiatry 1991;48:633–642.
38 Faraone SV, Biederman J, Mennin D, et al: Attention-deficit hyperactivity disorder with bipolar disorder: a familial subtype? J Am Acad Child Adolesc Psychiatry 1997;36:1378–1387.
39 Faraone SV, Biederman J, Jetton JG, Tsuang MT: Attention deficit disorder and conduct disorder: longitudinal evidence for a familial subtype. Psychol Med 1997;27:291–300.
40 Braaten EB, Biederman J, Monuteaux MC, Mick E, Calhoun E, Cattan G, Faraone SV: Revisiting the association between attention-deficit/hyperactivity disorder and anxiety disorders: a familial risk analysis. Biol Psychiatry 2003;53:93–99.
41 Goodman R, Stevenson J: A twin study of hyperactivity. II. The etiological role of genes, family relationships, and perinatal adversity. J Child Psychol Psychiatry 1989;30:691–709.
42 Sherman DK, McGue MK, Iacono WG: Twin concordance for attention deficit hyperactivity disorder: a comparison of teachers' and mothers' reports. Am J Psychiatry 1997;154:532–535.
43 Levy F, Hay DA, McStephen M, Wood C, Waldman I: Attention-deficit hyperactivity disorder: a category or a continuum? Genetic analysis of a large-scale twin study. Am Acad Child Adolesc Psychiatry 1997;36:737–744.
44 Hudziak JJ, Rudiger LP, Neale MC, et al: A twin study of inattentive, aggressive, and anxious/depressed behaviors. Am Acad Child Adolesc Psychiatry 2000;39:469–476.
45 Safer DJ: A familial factor in minimal brain dysfunction. Behav Genet 1973;3:175–186.
46 Cantwell DP: Genetic studies of hyperactive children: psychiatric illness in biological and adopting parents; in Fieve R, Rosenthal D, Brill H (eds): Genetic Research in Psychiatry. Baltimore, John Hopkins University Press, 1975.
47 Deutsch CK: PhD Dissertation. The University of Texas at Austin, 1983.
48 Shastry BS: Molecular genetics of attention-deficit hyperactivity disorder: an update. Neurochem Int 2004;44:469–474.
49 Faraone SV, Khan SA: Candidate gene studies of attention-deficit/hyperactivity disorder. J Clin Psychiatry 2006;67(suppl 8):13–20.
50 Reimherr FW, Wender PH, Ebert MH, Wood DR: Cerebrospinal fluid homovanillic acid and 5-hydroxyindoleacetic acid in adults with attention deficit disorder, residual type. Psychiatry Res 1984;11:71–78.
51 Shetty T, Chase TN: Central monoamines and hyperkinesis of childhood. Neurology 1976;26:1000–1002.
52 Shaywitz BA, Cohen DJ, Bowers MB: CSF monoamine metabolites in children with minimal brain dysfunction: evidence for alteration in of brain dopamine. J Pediatr 1977;7:90:67–71.
53 Reimherr FW, Wender PH, Wood DR, et al: An open trial of L-tyrosine in the treatment of attention deficit disorder, residual type. Am J Psychiatry 1987; 144:1071–1073.
54 Wood DR, Reimherr FW, Wender PH: Effects of levodopa on attention deficit disorder, residual type. Psychiatry Res 1982;6:13–20.
55 Wender PH, Wood DR, Reimherr FW, et al: An open trial of pargyline in the treatment of attention deficit disorder, residual type. Psychiatry Res 1983; 9:329–336
56 Wood DR, Reimherr FW, Wender PH, et al: Diagnosis and treatment of minimal brain dysfunction in adults. Arch Gen Psychiatry 1976;3:1453–1460.
57 Wender PH, Reimherr FW, Wood D, et al: A controlled study of methylphenidate in the treatment of attention deficit disorder, residual type. Am J Psychiatry 1985;142:547–552.

58 Wender PH, Reimherr FW: Bupropion treatment of attention-deficit hyperactivity disorder in adults. Am J Psychiatry 1990;147:1018–1020.
59 Wood DR, Reimherr FW, Wender PH: Treatment of attention deficit disorder with D,L-phenylalanine. Psychiatry Res 1985;16:21–26.
60 Wender PH, Reimherr FW: Bupropion treatment of attention-deficit hyperactivity disorder in adults. Am J Psychiatry 1990;147:1018–1020.
61 Wilens TE, Spencer TJ, Biederman J, et al: A controlled clinical trial of bupropion for attention deficit hyperactivity disorder in adults. Am J Psychiatry 2001;158:282–288.
62 Wilens TE, Haight BR, Horrigan JP, et al: Bupropion XL in adults with attention-deficit/hyperactivity disorder: a randomized, placebo-controlled study. Biol Psychiatry 2005;57:793–801.
63 Reimherr FW, Marchant BK, Strong RE, et al: Emotional dysregulation in adult ADHD and response to atomoxetine. Biol Psychiatry 2005;58:125–131.
64 Biederman J, Swanson JM, Wigal SB, et al: A comparison of once-daily and divided doses of modafinil in children with attention-deficit/hyperactivity disorder: a randomized, double-blind, and placebo-controlled study. J Clin Psychiatry 2006;67:727–735.
65 Mattes JA, Boswell L, Oliver H: Methylphenidate effects on symptoms of attention deficit disorder in adults. Arch Gen Psychiatry 1984;41:1059–1063.
66 Spencer T, Wilens T, Biederman J, et al: A double-blind, crossover comparison of methylphenidate and placebo in adults with childhood-onset attention-deficit hyperactivity disorder. Arch Gen Psychiatry 1995;52:434–443.
67 Spencer T, Biederman J, Wilens T, et al: A large, double-blind, randomized clinical trial of methylphenidate in the treatment of adults with attention-deficit/hyperactivity disorder. Biol Psychiatry 2005;57:456–463.
68 Rösler M, Fischer R, Ammer R, Ose C, Retz W, on behalf of the study group: A randomised, placebo-controlled, 24-week, study of low-dose extended-release methylphenidate in adults with attention-deficit/hyperactivity disorder. Eur Arch Psychiatry Clin Neurosci 2009;259:120–129.
69 Wender PH: Pharmacotherapy of attention-.deficit/hyperactivity disorder in adults. J Clin Psychiatry 1998;59(suppl 17):76–79.

Appendix A

Parents' rating scale: To be filled out by the mother of the subject (or father only if mother is unavailable).

Instructions: Listed below are items concerning children's behavior and the problems they sometimes have. Read each item carefully and decide how much you think your child was bothered by these problems when he/she was between 6 and 10 years old. Rate the amount of the problem by putting a check in the column that describes your child at that time.

	Not at all	Just a little	Pretty much	Very much
1. Restless (overactive)				
2. Excitable, impulsive				
3. Disturbs other children				
4. Fails to finish things started (short attention span)				
5. Fidgeting				
6. Inattentive, distractible				
7. Demands must be met immediately; gets frustrated				
8. Cries				
9. Mood changes quickly				
10. Temper outbursts (explosive and unpredictable behavior)				

Appendix B

Wender Utah Rating Scale: WURS scoring template: assign values (0–4 as indicated) to the 25 items shaded. Add scores. Scores of 41 or greater indicate probability that an adult had ADHD in childhood.

As a child I was (or had):	0	1	2	3	4
	Not at all or very slightly	Mildly	Moder-ately	Quite a bit	Very much
1. Active, restless, always on the go					
2. Afraid of things					
3. Concentration problems, easily distracted					
4. Anxious, worrying					
5. Nervous, fidgety					
6. Inattentive, daydreaming					
7. Hot- or short-tempered, low boiling point					
8. Shy, sensitive					
9. Temper outbursts, tantrums					

Appendix B. Continued

As a child I was (or had):	0 Not at all or very slightly	1 Mildly	2 Moder-ately	3 Quite a bit	4 Very much
10. Trouble with stick-to-it-iveness, not following through to finish things started					
11. Stubborn, strong-willed					
12. Sad or blue, depressed, unhappy					
13. Incautious, dare-devilish, involved in pranks					
14. Not getting a kick out of things, dissatisfied with life					
15. Disobedient with parents, rebellious, sassy					
16. Low opinion of myself					
17. Irritable					
18. Outgoing, friendly, enjoy company of people					
19. Sloppy, disorganized					
20. Moody, ups and downs					
21. Angry					
22. Friendly, popular					
23. Well-organized, tidy, neat					
24. Acting without thinking, impulsive					
25. Tendency to be immature					
26. Guilty feelings, regretful					
27. Losing control of myself					
28. Tendency to be or act irrational					
29. Unpopular with other children, didn't keep friends for long, didn't get along with other children					
30. Poorly coordinated did not participate in sports					
31. Afraid of losing control of self					
32. Well-coordinated, picked first in games					

Appendix B. Continued

As a child I was (or had):	0 Not at all or very slightly	1 Mildly	2 Moder-ately	3 Quite a bit	4 Very much
33. Tomboyish (for women only)					
34. Running away from home					
35. Getting into fights					
36. Teasing other children					
37. Leader, bossy					
38. Difficulty getting awake					
39. Follower, led around too much					
40. Trouble seeing things from someone else's point of view					
41. Trouble with authorities trouble with school; visits to principals office					
42. Trouble with police, booked, convicted					

Appendix B. Continued

Medical problems as a child:	0 Not at all or very slightly	1 Mildly	2 Moder ately	3 Quite a bit	4 Very much
43. Headache					
44. Stomach aches					
45. Constipation					
46. Diarrhea					
47. Food allergies					
48. Other allergies					
49. Bedwetting					

Appendix B. Continued

As a child in school, I was (or had):	0 Not at all or very slightly	1 Mildly	2 Moder-ately	3 Quite a bit	4 Very much
50. Overall, a good student, fast					
51. Overall, a poor student, slow learner					
52. Slow in learning to read					
53. Slow reader					
54. Trouble reversing letters					
55. Problems with spelling					
56. Trouble with mathematics or numbers					
57. Bad handwriting					
58. Able to read pretty well, but never really enjoyed reading					
59. Not achieving up to potential					
60. Repeating grades (which grades?)					
61. Suspended or expelled (which grades?)					

Appendix C

Wender-Reimherr Adult Attention Deficit Disorder Scale (WRAADDS), May 2003

Subject Identification: .... Date: .... Rater: ....

This interview is intended to measure the severity of the seven target symptoms of the Utah Criteria in adults who have been diagnosed with Attention Deficit Hyperactivity Disorder (ADHD). The scale is not intended to diagnose ADHD. Clearly, all of these symptoms occur in other psychiatric disorders and this scale is useful only when other disorders have been assessed. The symptoms should be present chronically although they may be aggravated by stress.

The scale is most valid when obtained during a joint interview with the subject and a cooperative informant such as a partner, parent or sibling.

Appendix C. Continued

The individual questions should be followed by general probes:

How much (often, long, severe) has this occurred?
Have others commented about this?
What have they said?
What difficulties or problems has this caused with other people, work or school?

The individual items should be rated as follows:

0 – None, not present
1 – Mild, somewhat or sometimes true
2 – Clearly present or often true

The summary scores should be based on the ratings of the specific questions, together with any other symptoms in the area reported by the subject. The summary score should not be a simple average of the individual ratings. If only one question group is rated as clearly present, a rating of '4' might be appropriate if this one factor is causing significant problems. A total score suggesting of ADHD is considered by the authors to be >18, although there is no data and it is the user's decision.

Summary Ratings:

0 – None
1 – Mild
2 – Moderate
3 – Quite a bit
4 – Very much

Wender-Reimherr Adult Attention Deficit Disorder Scale (WRAADDS), May 2003

Subject Identification: .... Date: .... Rater: ....

1. Attention Difficulties: **Summary Rating 0–4** ....

Do you have difficulties keeping your attention on things, concentrating, focusing?	0	1	2
Do you have problems with your mind wandering?			

Appendix C. Continued

Are you easily distracted? Do you have problems concentrating if sounds or any other distractions are present?	0	1	2
Do you have difficulty keeping your mind on conversations? Do others complain that you do not listen, that you don't pay attention to them when they're talking?	0	1	2
In formal settings such as classes, meetings, church, programs or lectures, do you have difficulty paying attention to the speaker? (Do not rate this item if the subject does not engage in these activities.)	0	1	2
Do you have difficulty keeping your mind on reading? Do you avoid or dislike reading anything which is not of special interest? Do you frequently have to re-read because your mind drifts off, or do you have difficulty comprehending written material?	0	1	2
2. Hyperactivity/Restlessness: **Summary Rating 0–4**			
Do you have difficulty relaxing? Do you often feel restless or tense?	0	1	2
Are you overactive; do you prefer to be always on the go? Do you have difficulty remaining seated at work, school, or home? Do you have to get up and move around frequently? Are you unable to sit through a movie or TV show?	0	1	2
Are you fidgety? Do people notice that you are fidgety? Do you have difficulty sitting still; do you frequently shift your position? Do you drum your fingers, play with things, move your legs, bite your nails, twirl your hair or tap your feet? (either by report or observation)	0	1	2

3. Temper: **Summary Rating 0–4** ....

Do you frequently feel irritable or angry with your spouse, children, or other family members or at work, driving, or in other situations?	0	1	2
Do you have angry outbursts or lose your temper easily? Do you have a 'short fuse' or a 'low boiling point'?	0	1	2
Does your temper cause problems for you? Do you lose control during temper outbursts? (saying things you regret, becoming aggressive, acting in a threatening manner, or behaving impulsively)	0	1	2

4. Affective Lability: **Summary Rating 0–4** ....

Prior to scoring this question, the rater must differentiate between a major mood disorder and the lability of mood in subjects with ADHD. ADHD-related dysphoria is generally brief, lasting hours, and usually has an identifiable precipitant. The exception is when the subject experiences persistent life problems (often self-produced), when the period of dysphoria may be extended. Similarly, distinguish between excitement (which may be mild) and overenthusiasm from mood elevation with a manic quality.

ADHD subjects may be comorbid for a major depression. Determine duration and frequency of episodes and presence of somatic concomitants to help distinguish discouragement, moodiness, and demoralization found in ADHD from major depression with its loss of interest and loss of the ability to experience pleasure.

Does your mood change frequently, going up and down – like a roller coaster in the sense of getting sad or feeling 'up'?	0	1	2
Do you often have periods of being sad, blue, or discouraged? During these periods, are you overly self-critical or down on yourself?	0	1	2
Do you often feel bored? Do you easily lose interest in things?	0	1	2

Appendix C. Continued

Do you have periods of being excessively active, hyper, getting too excited, going too fast, or talking too much?	0	1	2
5. Emotional Overreactivity: **Summary Rating 0–4**			
Do you easily get feelings of being overwhelmed? Do you frequently feel 'hassled', frustrated?	0	1	2
Do you overreact to pressure, blow things out of proportion? Do small problems seem too difficult; do you 'make mountains out of molehills'?	0	1	2
When these reactions occur, do you have difficulties in managing tasks or getting things done? With pressures or stresses, do you become anxious, disorganized or confused?	0	1	2
6. Disorganization: **Summary Rating 0–4**			
Do you have problems with organization at home, work or school? Do you have difficulties organizing your time, setting priorities, working in an organized manner?	0	1	2
Do you jump from one task to another before finishing the first? Do you have trouble 'with stick-to-it-ive-ness'? Do you start projects, but have trouble staying with them to completion?	0	1	2
Are you forgetful? Do you forget to return phone calls or to keep appointments? Do you frequently misplace things like keys, purse, wallet, or things around the house or at work?	0	1	2

Appendix C. Continued

Do you have problems getting started, putting things off, procrastinating? Do you put off everything to the last minute? Do you have trouble meeting deadlines?	0	1	2
7. Impulsivity: **Summary Rating 0–4**			
Do you have problems with being impulsive? Do you frequently jump into things without thinking? Do you make sudden decisions without thinking?	0	1	2
Are you impulsive in talking? Do you interrupt others? Do you finish sentences for others? Do you say things without thinking, or blurt things out? Do you frequently regret what you have said?	0	1	2
Are you impulsive with money? Do you impulse buy or have trouble managing money?	0	1	2
Do you rush through activities or work, try to do things too quickly? Do you frequently ignore details? Do you make careless mistakes?	0	1	2
Are you impatient, or unable to wait? Do others regard you as impatient (friends, family)?	0	1	2
Total Score (sum of 7 summary items):			

Prof. David A. Tomb, MD
Department of Psychiatry, University of Utah School of Medicine
Salt Lake City, UT 84132 (USA)
E-Mail David.Tomb@m.cc.utah.edu

Retz W, Klein RG (eds): Attention-Deficit Hyperactivity Disorder (ADHD) in Adults.
Key Issues in Mental Health. Basel, Karger, 2010, vol 176, pp 38–57

Family and Twin Studies in Attention-Deficit Hyperactivity Disorder

Christine Margarete Freitag[a] · Wolfgang Retz[b]

[a]Department of Child and Adolescent Psychiatry, Frankfurt University Hospital, Frankfurt, and [b]Institute for Forensic Psychology and Psychiatry, Saarland University Hospital, Homburg/Saar, Germany

Abstract

Twin and family studies in attention-deficit hyperactivity disorder (ADHD) did result in the findings of a strong heritable component (60–80%) of this disorder in children and adolescents. Twin studies have not yet been performed in adults. In addition to increased rates of ADHD in parents and siblings of children with ADHD, family studies resulted in a high risk for ADHD in the offspring of parents with ADHD implying strong familial, i.e. genetic or environmental risk factors in the adult form. This corroborates findings from twin studies, which suggested that persistent ADHD might be an interesting phenotype for molecular genetic studies. The present review thoroughly presents findings from twin and family studies with regard to ADHD subtypes, sex differences, comorbidity rates, diagnostic aspects and environmental influences on ADHD. Besides persistent ADHD, ADHD with symptoms of conduct disorder or antisocial personality disorder might be another strongly genetically determined subtype, however family environmental risk factors have also been established for this pattern of comorbidity.

All psychiatric disorders are environmentally as well as genetically determined. To quantify the impact of these different factors on disease status or disease severity, family and twin studies are performed. These studies either estimate concordance rates of disease status in families or in monozygotic (MZ) and dizygotic twins (DZ) or the heritability of a disorder, i.e. the phenotypic variation due to additive genetic effects. Family studies allow to estimate a recurrence risk for the disorder, which can be translated into a heritability estimate, and additionally may allow to elicit a certain pattern of inheritance, if the disorder of interest seems to be a mendelian disorder. Heritability estimates as well as the quantification of shared and non-shared environmental effects in twin studies are obtained by a comparison of the phenotypic variance within and between MZ and DZ twin pairs. Studies on twins reared apart or adoption studies are other designs to assess the influence of genetic and environmental risk factors. Estimation of genetic and environmental effects on the disorder in these studies is based on the assumption of random mating, absence of gene-gene and gene-environment interaction and unlinked loci.

In attention-deficit hyperactivity disorder (ADHD) most family and twin studies have been performed in children and adolescents, and not in adults. This mainly has been due to the diagnostic difficulties encountered in adult ADHD (see chapter 3) and in the past also due to a limited recognition of the disorder in adults. This chapter, therefore, differentially reports results of family and twin studies in children and adolescents as well as of family studies in adults. It further discusses the stability of environmental and genetic influences over the lifespan on disease status or disease severity as well as on rates of comorbidity (also see chapter 4).

Twin Studies

The earliest twin study on the heritability of hyperactivity was performed by Willerman [1] in 1973. This study, however, used a volunteer sample and questionnaires of uncertain validity. Due to the nature of the variance components method used to assess heritability, a volunteer sample might falsify results, because the more equal the environment the stronger the calculated genetic effects and vice versa. The first representative twin study, which assessed ADHD symptoms by the Rutter teacher and parent questionnaires, found that genetic effects accounted for around 75% of the explainable variance of hyperactivity and attention difficulties [2, 3]. Since then, numerous twin studies in children and adolescents have been performed, and the finding of a heritable component of about 60–80% [4] was replicated in different populations, however mainly of Caucasian origin. These heritability estimates were independent of age and sex distribution of the twin samples. Several issues as the definition of ADHD as category or continuum, subtypes within ADHD, assessment instruments, differential effects of informants or rater contrast, sex differences, comorbidity rates, environmental risk factors, and the impact of genetic and environmental risk factors on the course of the disorder were additionally addressed. Only one twin study in adults has been performed to date, which assessed the efficacy of retrospective recall of ADHD symptoms in adults around age 50 years [5].

Categorical Diagnosis or Continuously Distributed Trait

Differing from family studies, which often obtained categorical diagnoses and compared rates of disorders in relatives, most twin studies were based on rating scales, resulting in a continuously distributed measure of ADHD symptoms in the study population. The study by Levy et al. [6] compared heritability estimates obtained either by continuous or categorical data, and also estimated heritability by sibling data. A rating scale based on DSM-III-R diagnostic criteria as well as a structured diagnostic interview was used. Definition of ADHD by continuous or categorical data as well as familial relationship did not change the resulting estimates of an additive genetic effect in the range of 75–90%. This finding is supportive of a continuously underlying trait, which most likely is mediated by several genes. Therefore, ADHD might be conceptualized as an oligogenic or polygenic disorder. The concordance rate <100% in MZ twins, however, also implies environmental effects in ADHD.

Another study [7] found a heritability of 89% by comparing concordance rates (categorical diagnoses) obtained through a structured interview with the mother, and a heritability of 73% by categorical diagnoses obtained through teacher questionnaires. Combined mother and teacher data resulted in a heritability estimate of 79%. This points to differential reporter or rater effects (see below). It can be concluded that categorical or continuous measurements did result in comparable heritability estimates for childhood ADHD from twin studies.

The above-mentioned and other twin studies [8–10] assessed attention and hyperactivity/impulsivity symptoms together. In DSM-IV [11], however, the inattentive subtype has become a separate diagnosis from the hyperactive/impulsive subtype and the combined disorder. This has posed, first, the question of heritability of the respective subtypes and, second, of shared genetic factors underlying these subtypes.

Heritability of ADHD Subtypes

The heritability of attention difficulties as measured by the Child Behavior Checklist (CBCL), a parent questionnaire [12], was assessed by several twin studies [13–16]. Estimates of heritability of attention problems lay around 70–80%, with non-shared environmental influences accounting for the remaining variance. The CBCL, however, does not contain the same attention items as DSM-IV or DSM-III-R. Therefore, it was necessary to replicate these findings for attention difficulties as assessed by DSM-III-R or DSM-IV criteria.

In boys, one study [17] did show far lower heritability estimates for attention difficulties due to DSM-III-R criteria as rated by teachers (39%) compared to mothers (69%). The hyperactivity/impulsivity subtype, which was also assessed in this study, was found to show a higher heritability, both in teacher (69%) and mother ratings (91%). The same study found that common genetic factors might influence both subtypes, however, again teacher ratings (33%) and mother ratings (86%) did differ considerably. These findings again are indicative of rater effects, which can confound heritability estimates (see below).

Still, the study shows stronger genetic influences on hyperactivity/impulsivity symptoms than on attention problems. Strong genetic influences on hyperactivity symptoms as assessed by the Rutter A scale as well as indication of a rater-contrast effect were also observed in two other twin studies [18, 19].

A further study in 8- to 16-year-old twins [9] assessed the three dimensions inattention, hyperactivity and impulsivity separately at two different time points. In contrast to the above-mentioned study, data were indicative of a differential genetic determination of inattention as compared to hyperactivity and impulsivity, the latter, however, sharing the same genetic risk factors. Similar results had been obtained in the analysis of a bigger set of twin data from the same study at only one time point [20]. In the latter study, additionally multiple measures of ADHD symptomatology were compared, i.e. an investigator-based interview, the Rutter parent and teacher questionnaires and the CBCL. Maternal measures indicated that on the phenotypic level the different measurement instruments assessed the same underlying behavioral construct for inattention, hyperactivity and impulsivity problems respectively. Again, rater-specific variance was found for both parent and teacher data.

Another approach assessing subtypes has been data-driven. These studies first established the latent class structure of DSM-IV symptoms in population-based samples of twins to parse individuals empirically into subtypes on a purely statistical, i.e. probabilistic, level. Second, concordance rates or recurrence risk in MZ and DZ twins were compared to differentially assess the genetic background of each subtype. DSM-IV symptoms were obtained by mother/parent ratings only. Studies across cultures (USA and Australia) elicited 8 subtypes, of which 3 were severe classes (severe inattentive, severe combined, severe hyperactive/impulsive) which roughly correspond to the DSM-IV-based subtypes. The other 5 classes consisted of individuals with mild inattentive, mild hyperactive/impulsive or mild combined symptoms, which did not reach diagnostic criteria according to DSM-IV. The few symptom class was comprised of unaffected individuals. One symptom pattern emerged which is not covered by DSM-IV, a talkative-impulsive subtype [21–24]. Differences between MZ and DZ in either concordance rates or recurrence risks were found for the 3 severe and the 3 mild classes as well as for the talkative-impulsive subtype, with strongest genetic influences on the severe inattentive and the severe hyperactive-impulsive subtypes [24, 25]. Cross-subtype recurrence risks were far lower. These studies, therefore, are supportive of the DSM-IV distinction of attention-deficit, hyperactivity-impulsivity and the combined ADHD and its relevance for genetic studies. Further, they also support the continuous trait model of ADHD. As the mild and severe combined type did show a smaller recurrence risk ratio than the severe inattentive and severe hyperactive-impulsive subtypes, they also indicate a differential genetic determination of attention difficulties and other symptoms in ADHD.

In conclusion, there is some inconsistency between studies regarding the amount of genetic influences on attention problems. The studies agree with regard to a prevailing differential genetic determination of attention problems and hyperactive-impulsive symptoms, however with some genetic overlap between symptoms.

Rater Effects

The above-mentioned studies assessed ADHD symptoms by parental and/or teacher questionnaires. Informant-specific ratings were obtained in almost all studies, with considerable varying heritability estimates, when only parental (typically, maternal), teacher or combined ratings were taken into account [7, 8, 17, 26–28]. In most studies, mothers did show a rater-contrast effect by rating the child with high ADHD symptoms higher, and the child with low ADHD symptoms less severely than the teacher, making 'true' differences in behavior unlikely [26]. These rater-contrast effects, however, might also be measurement-specific, as studies assessing ADHD symptoms by the Rutter A scale or the DuPaul ADHD scale did show a stronger difference between DZ twins, indicating rater-contrast effects, than studies using other measurement instruments [6, 14, 20, 27, 29, 30]. Interestingly, a study using the Strengths and Weaknesses of ADHD-Symptoms and Normal-Behavior (SWAN) scale as parent rating scale, which includes above-average performance on attention and activity, resulted in higher DZ twin concordance and lower variability in DZ measurements, implying less rater-contrast effect for this scale [31]. If due to rater-contrast effects variability between DZ twins is estimated higher and concordance lower than between MZ twins, this will result in an overestimation of heritability and underestimation of environmental effects as well as in contradicting results with respect to the impact of shared and non-shared environmental influences on the disorder. On the contrary, the same teacher in one study tended to rate twin pairs in general more similar than different teachers, resulting in a possible underestimation of heritability [26].

In addition to rater-contrast effects, several studies have shown that agreement between mothers/parents and teachers or between teachers on corresponding ADHD scales generally is quite low (e.g. Sherman et al. [17]: r = 0.3 parent-teacher; Simonoff et al. [26]: r = 0.5 teacher-teacher; Thapar et al. [27]: r = 0.4 parent-teacher). This points towards the possibility that mothers/parent and teacher questionnaires might assess somewhat differing pathology. Due to this problem, attempts have been made to utilize pervasive ADHD, i.e. the categorical diagnosis obtained by mother/parent as well as teacher reports simultaneously as phenotype in molecular genetic studies to avoid inclusion of phenocopies of the disorder and to improve power of genetic association studies. It has been shown that the pervasive subtype is as heritable as the mother/parent-rated ADHD, and in some studies has shown a better predictive validity than ADHD as defined by mother/parent or teacher ratings only [20, 28, 32].

Sex Effects

The above-mentioned studies were performed in female and male children and adolescents. As the sex difference in prevalence estimates of ADHD is about 3:1 with slightly higher rates of the combined type in male individuals and slightly lower sex differences for the inattentive subtype [33, 34], twin studies have also been analyzed with regard to differing genetic and environmental effects in female and male twins. No effects of sex on heritability estimates regarding the three subtypes and only small differences in environmental effects regarding shared and non-shared environmental factors were detected. However, the pattern of associated comorbidities (see below) did differ [9, 10, 35, 36]. One study found higher rates of ADHD symptoms in the DZ co-twins or siblings of girls with ADHD compared to boys with ADHD, indicative of a polygenic multiple threshold model [37].

Comorbidity of ADHD

In children with ADHD, high rates of comorbidity are found. In a population-based sample of twins aged 8–18 years, around 70% of the children with the inattentive or the hyperactive/impulsive subtype and around 90% of the children with the combined subtype did show at least one comorbid disorder [38]. The most prevalent comorbid disorders were Oppositional Defiant Disorder (ODD; 40–65%), Conduct Disorder (CD; 27–47%), Major Depressive Disorder (MDD; 0–24%) and Generalized Anxiety Disorder (GAD; 13–21%), similar to rates estimated from epidemiological studies [39]. ODD and CD were higher in the combined ADHD subtype only (ODD: 66%; CD: 47%), whereas MDD was associated with the inattentive (24%) and the combined subtypes (22%). Another frequent comorbidity of ADHD is reading disability (RD; around 40%), which in most studies did show a stronger association with attention problems than with hyperactive/impulsive symptoms [39–42].

Regarding the etiology of the comorbid symptoms and disorders, most studies on RD and ADHD agree with respect to common genetic factors influencing RD and inattention [43]. All of these studies used mother/parent reported problems only. In the study by Willcutt et al. [34], about 95% of the phenotypic covariance between RD symptoms of inattention was attributable to common genetic influences, whereas only 21% of the phenotypic overlap between RD and hyperactivity/impulsivity was due to the same genetic factors.

Epidemiological twin studies on maternally/paternally rated comorbidity of ADHD and ODD or CD elicited sex differences with regard to ODD/CD symptom severity with more ODD/CD symptoms in males [18]. A study in 7- to 13-year-old twins, adjusted for rater-contrast effects [36], found ODD/CD symptoms in males to be more strongly genetically determined that in females (heritability males: 66%, females: 50%). Covariation of ADHD and ODD/CD symptoms, however, did not show differences between females and males and implicated a common genetic factor underlying the comorbidity of ADHD and ODD/CD symptoms. About 50% of the additive genetic effects were shared between ADHD and ODD/CD as well as about 40% of the unique environmental effects. Interestingly, with regard to ODD/CD symptoms, no rater-contrast effects were found, contrary to the findings in ADHD. Similar findings were obtained in 5- to 17-year-old twins with or without comorbid CD symptoms. Heritability estimates for CD symptoms lay around 50%, and common genetic influences were postulated for ADHD and CD, indicating a genetically more extreme variant of ADHD [44]. However, additional shared and non-shared environmental influences were found for CD only.

Simultaneous analysis of teacher and parent/mother questionnaires obtained on 8- to 16-year-old twins did result in slightly different findings: no sex differences in heritability for ODD/CD were found, and the genetic correlation between ADHD and CD symptoms was higher (64–82%) [9]. Again, substantial environmental effects were found for ODD/CD only. Further, inattention was influenced by a different genetic factor than hyperactivity/impulsivity, and this factor also did influence the comorbidity of inattention and ODD/CD.

A further study assessed covariation among childhood externalizing disorders by interviews with the 14-year-old twins themselves [45]. Again, covariation among the three disorders ADHD, ODD and CD was attributed to shared genetic influence on the disorders as well as to non-shared environmental influences. For each disorder in this study, however, also some unique environmental influences were found.

Contrary to the above reported findings, a study in 11-year-old twins found a single shared environmental factor most strongly contributing to the covariation of ADHD, ODD and CD symptoms [46]. A bigger sample from the same study was analyzed differently to also assess informant effects, as in the study child and mother interview data were obtained. In males, higher self and mother reported ADHD, ODD and CD symptoms were found than in females. Correlations of mother and child reports were around 25% [47].

Self-reports resulted in less genetic influence on the three disorders as well as in different patterns of correlations between disorders compared to the mother data implying a shared environmental factor underlying the three disorders. Analysis of mother data, on the contrary, resulted in a strong genetic factor underlying the comorbidity of the three disorders.

In conclusion, studies do not agree with regard to genetic and environmental mediation of the high rate of comorbidity of ADHD with ODD or CD. The different findings might be due to the lack of distinction of ODD and CD in some studies (see below, section on family studies), to age differences between samples or to the differing measurement instruments used. As child report data do show a limited reliability and validity regarding externalizing disorders compared to parent/mother or teacher reports [48], the findings obtained from studies relying strongly on child report data should be viewed with some caution. Concluding from parent and teacher data, common genetic and non-shared environmental effects seem to influence the comorbidity of ADHD, ODD and CD, however additional genetic and environmental risk factors specific for each disorder cannot be excluded.

The impact of genetic or environmental influences on comorbidity rates of ADHD with MDD and anxiety disorders has rarely been studied in twin samples. In one study, using the latent class approach assessing information on separation anxiety, ODD and depression as well as ADHD symptoms by parent or child report in a sample of female twins aged 13–23 years, 9 latent classes emerged, of which 2 were 'comorbid' types, i.e. ADHD inattentive subtype + ODD and ADHD combined subtype + ODD for which heritability estimates of 63 and 81% were obtained. The ADHD combined subtype + ODD latent class comprised additional depression and anxiety items, which might be specific for a female sample [49]. These results support the previously mentioned studies with regard to common genetic as well as environmental effects underlying comorbid ADHD and ODD. No specific additional genetic effects for comorbid MDD or anxiety were detected.

Stability of Genetic and Environmental Influences on Lifespan

Longitudinal twin studies have been performed to assess the stability of ADHD diagnosis, subtype and comorbid ODD/CD to elicit genetic and environmental influences on stability and change. Three studies assessed the stability of ADHD symptoms. In the first study, twins were assessed for DSM-III-R-based ADHD symptoms at age 8–9 years old and reassessed 5 years later [50]. Heritability at the first assessment was 68% for girls and only 35% for boys, whereas at the second assessment, it was 61% for girls and 74% for boys. Genetic and non-shared environmental effects were important for stability as well as for change. Due to the low heritability estimates obtained at wave I for boys in this study, however, these results have to be viewed with caution. In a sample of younger twins aged 2, 3, and 4 years, assessing only 4 ADHD symptoms rated by mothers/parents, a phenotypic correlation of around 50% over the years was elicited [51]. Heritability at age 2, 3, and 4 was estimated around 80% with non-shared environmental influences accounting for the remaining variance. Continuity of ADHD symptoms in this study was mediated 91% by additive genetic influences. The same sample was assessed at age 7 and 8 years by the Strengths and Difficulties Questionnaire and the Conners' Rating Scales obtained from mothers/parents [29]. In the univariate analysis at age 8 years, in addition to additive genetic (72%) and non-shared environmental factors (14%), also shared environmental risk factors (14%) were found. Phenotypic correlation across time points 2, 3, 4, 7, and 8 years old were mediated by shared genetic influences (59–96%) and child-specific environmental influences the latter of which also accounted for change in behavior.

A third study assessed stability and change of CBCL derived Overactivity (OA) and Attention Problems (AP) in 3-, 7-, 10-, and 12-year-old twins [52]. The older the children, the more stable AP became in the individual. Across ages, additive and dominant genetic effects did influence the stability of AP (around 70%). 30% of the residual variance was explained by non-shared environmental effects. In this study, rater-contrast effects were not controlled for which might have resulted in an overestimation of genetic effects on the stability of symptoms.

One study has been performed which assessed the ADHD hyperactivity/impulsivity and inattention subtypes according to DSM-III and/or DSM-IV symptoms separately at three time points (age 8–9, 13–14, and 16–17 years old; sample of Larsson et al. [50]). Cross-type correlations were as high as subtype-specific correlations. 45–90% of the total genetic variance in each measure was explained by persistent genetic influences. However, in most cases, persistent cross-subtype influences explained more genetic variance than persistent subtype-specific influences. Additionally, age-specific genetic effects were present. Results were interpreted with regard to strongest persistent genetic influences on the ADHD combined type with some support of differential genetic influences on the hyperactive/impulsive and inattentive subtypes. Furthermore, age-limited genetic effects suggested genetic contributions to changes in symptoms of ADHD. The remaining variance again was explained by non-shared environmental effects.

Taken together, from childhood to adolescence, persisting combined ADHD as well as inattention seem to be influenced strongly by genetic effects and to a lesser extent by non-shared environmental effects. Therefore, persistent ADHD might be an interesting phenotype for molecular genetic studies. This also can be expected from ADHD persisting into adulthood. However, the problem of recall bias [5] as well as missing parental information on pregnancy and early development might lead to an increased rate of false-positive or false-negative diagnoses in adults with suspected ADHD reducing the power of molecular genetic studies.

Only one study has assessed the genetic structure underlying the persistence of ADHD and ODD/CD after 19 months in 8- to 16-year-old twins by mother and teacher rating scales [9]. Covariation among phenotypes across informants and over time were governed by a common set of genes, but not a single genetic factor. Substantial environmental effects were found for ODD/CD, but not for the covariation of ADHD and ODD/CD. The findings of this study are limited, as the sample comprised twins of a broad age range who were followed for a relatively short period. However, findings resemble the results of the cross-sectional studies, implying mainly genetic and to a lesser extent environmental risk factors for comorbid ADHD und ODD/CD as well as for their persistence. The genetic risk factors for comorbidity or persistence, however, might be distinct. Similar to persistent ADHD, ADHD with comorbid ODD/CD might be an interesting phenotype for molecular genetic studies in ADHD.

Family Studies

Resembling twin studies, family studies in ADHD have been performed since the 1980s [53, 54]. Compared to twin studies, family studies provide some advantages. They are performed on individuals with ADHD and their families, therefore excluding risk factors associated with twinning itself, e.g. low birth weight, prematurity etc. Low birth weight in one twin study has been found to strongly influence discordant hyperactivity symptoms in MZ twins [55], implying factors associated with low birth weight as either shared or non-shared environmental risk factors for ADHD. On the other hand, genetic and environmental influences cannot easily be singled out in family studies. An increase in familial recurrence risk might be due to genetic as well as environmental risk factors associated with the disorder. One environmental risk factor strongly associated with ADHD, replicated by epidemiological and twin studies, is maternal smoking during pregnancy [56–58]. Most family studies did not control for this risk factor, as it has been replicated only recently.

Adoption Studies

Adoption studies can prove both genetic and environmental influences on the disorder, however they are difficult to perform due to limited numbers of adopted children as well as difficulties assessing the biological parents of the adopted children. The adoption studies performed in individuals with ADHD either did not assess the biological parents of the adopted children with ADHD [59] or did not use standardized assessment of ADHD symptoms [60–62]. Also, maternal smoking during pregnancy and other risk factors were not controlled for. Therefore, the findings of these studies are limited, however all studies lent some support to the hypothesis that ADHD has a genetic component.

Segregation Studies
In addition to heritability estimates, family studies also allow to explore the mode of inheritance underlying the genetics of ADHD. Segregation analyzes in families of children with ADHD [63] were indicative of a single major gene with low penetrance in contrast to twin studies, which were indicative of a continuously underlying trait most likely mediated by several genes. To date, both models are still abundant, however, with the exception of some linkage studies [64] molecular genetic research is predominately based on the oligogenic/polygenic model with additional environmental risk factors for ADHD which is supported by most twin studies. In contrast to twin studies, the segregation study by Maher et al. [63] also implicated differential genetic effects in female and male individuals with ADHD. However, the study was based on a distinct clinical population, which limits the generalization of its results.

Family Studies in Children with ADHD
Family studies are performed to elicit the risk that an individual is affected, given that a relative is. Two measures are usually assessed. The recurrence risk is the conditional probability that a relative of a certain degree of relationship to an affected individual is also affected. An alternative measure is the relative risk, i.e. the increase in risk compared to the population prevalence, given that a relative is affected. Heritability estimates can be derived from family studies based on expected phenotypic correlation between relatives. Estimates of genetic and environmental effects on phenotypic measures can be obtained by comparing different relatives with regard to recurrence risk or phenotypic correlation. The latter has rarely been done in family studies on ADHD, as in clinical and epidemiological settings it is difficult to gather data from greater than first-degree relatives.

Rates of ADHD and Other Psychiatric Disorders in Siblings and Parents of Children with ADHD
The first family studies in hyperactive children assessed psychiatric disorders in parents [65–70]. Due to non-blind rating, non-standardized diagnoses, insufficient control for SES or inadequate control groups, the results of these studies have to be viewed with caution. A first study assessing psychopathology in parents and siblings according to DSM-III criteria by direct interview with the parents and controlling for

SES elicited higher rates of attention-deficit disorder (ADD, DSM-IIII), ODD and MDD in first-degree relatives of 6- to 17-year-old children with ADD (n = 21) compared to the first-degree relatives of healthy control children (n = 20) [53]. Not a single relative with bipolar disorder, mental retardation or pervasive developmental disorder was seen in children with ADD, whereas the rate of enuresis was non-significantly increased. In an enlarged sample (n = 73) with an additional psychiatric control group (n = 26) without ADD, first-degree relatives of children with ADD did show higher rates of ADD, any antisocial disorder (combined ODD, CD, antisocial personality disorder) and drug dependence than both control groups [87]. Anxiety disorders and MDD were increased in first-degree relatives of both, children with ADD and children with another psychiatric disorder. Despite the familial aggregation genetic and environmental effects cannot be fully differentiated from family studies. The latter study, however, did explore psychosocial risk factors (low social class and separation/divorce in the family of origin) which were equally distributed in families with and without ADD, rendering these factors unlikely causes of DSM-III ADD. Comparable results on increased rates of ADDH (equal to ADD in DSM-III) in parents of children with ADDH, ADDH+CD and CD but not in children with emotional disorder or control children were obtained in another family study using DSM-III-R criteria for ADDH [71]. Findings of increased rates of ADHD in parents and siblings of children with ADHD were replicated in several other studies on parents, siblings and one study on second-degree relatives of children with ADHD according to DSM-III-R or DSM-IV criteria [72–75].

Similar to twin studies, the following aspects were differentially addressed in family studies on ADHD: the validity and segregation of the DSM-IV defined subtypes inattention, hyperactivity/impulsivity and combined ADHD, sex differences, rates of comorbid disorders, and environmental risk factors associated with ADHD in children and adolescents.

ADHD Subtypes

Only a few family studies have been performed analyzing the familial transmission of the inattentive, combined and hyperactive/impulsive ADHD subtypes separately. A recent study provided an analysis on the pooled data of six studies, exploring the familial transmission of the inattentive and combined ADHD subtypes [76]. New data were analyzed in addition to data from two twin [6, 24] and three family studies [75, 77, 78]. Results were indicative of heterogeneity of the inattentive subtype, sharing some of its etiology with the combined type, however also including cases with non-shared etiology. Further, in boys, the two subtypes were more clearly distinguishable than in girls. With regard to the hyperactive/impulsive subtype, no clear conclusions can be drawn from the family studies, as it is the rarest subtype, and family studies therefore lacked the power to elucidate differences regarding this subtype. Only one study indicated specificity of this subtype [79]. Taken together, results from family and twin studies agree on implying a prevailing differential genetic determination of attention problems and hyperactive-impulsive symptoms, however, with some genetic overlap between symptoms.

Sex Differences

Contrary to the studies assessing subtypes, most studies assessing ADD according to DSM-III or DSM-III-R did not find any differences between girls and boys regarding ADD and other psychiatric disorders in first-degree relatives of children with ADD [73, 79]. Only one study found a higher rate of ADHD in parents of sibling pairs who both were affected by ADHD and one of whom was female compared to male sibling pairs only [78], which might be indicative of a multifactorial threshold model, also suggested by the findings of one twin study [80]. Another study focusing on families with a parent with antisocial personality disorder or with the index child showing comorbid conduct disorder found a higher risk for ADHD in the siblings of boys with ADHD+CD but not of girls with ADHD+CD according to DSM-III-R diagnoses [81]. In families without antisocial disorders, these sex differences were not found. Findings again corroborate the results of twin studies, indicating no sex differences with respect to combined ADHD, but differential genetic and/or environmental effects in girls and boys regarding ADHD comorbid with CD and possible differences regarding the DSM-IV inattentive subtype [76].

Comorbid Disorders in Siblings and Parents

A recent review of family studies suggested that family studies based on prevalence rates might have a limited ability to lead to correct conclusions regarding the causes of comorbidity [82]. This renders the results of the presented studies preliminary.

Few family studies have been performed to elucidate the familiality of ADHD versus ADHD comorbid with ODD or CD despite the findings of high rates of ODD, CD or antisocial personality disorder in first-degree relatives in the early family studies (see above). In a study based on DSM-III diagnoses, rates of ADD were increased in first-degree relatives of children with ADD, ADD+oppositional disorder (OD according to DSM-III) and ADD+CD [83]. Morbidity risk for ADD, however, was highest in relatives of children with ADD+CD, implying ADD+CD as a more severe phenotype of ADD, which also has been suggested from results of some twin studies. Antisocial personality disorder was highest in relatives of children with ADD+CD and ADD+OD. In several studies implementing DSM-III-R or DSM-IV criteria, first-degree relatives of children with ADHD+CD did show higher rates of depression, substance abuse and antisocial personality disorder than families of children with ADHD without CD, of which maternal depression and paternal antisocial personality disorder seem to be a specific risk factor for comorbid CD in the offspring [78, 84–87].

Despite higher rates of anxiety disorders in parents of children with ADHD [85, 88, 89] two studies implementing DSM-III or DSM-III-R diagnoses found an independent segregation of anxiety disorders and ADD/ADHD, implying differential risk factors for both types of disorders [90, 91]. Another study assessing anxiety disorders in parents of young children with ADHD with or without comorbid ODD/CD found increased rates of anxiety disorders in mothers of children with ADHD+CD compared to healthy control children diagnosed according to DSM-III-R criteria [85]. However, when results were adjusted for comorbid anxiety disorders in children, the association of child ADHD+CD with anxiety disorder in the mother disappeared, again implying differential risk factors for both types of disorder.

With regard to MDD in parents of children with ADD, one early study implementing DSM-III criteria found an independent segregation of ADD and MDD [92]. More recent studies using DSM-III or DSM-III-R criteria, however, found some support for a familial link of ADHD and depression, which was most pronounced in ADHD families with antisocial disorders [85, 93–95]. Similarly, in several studies rates of ADHD in children of depressed parents were higher than in children of control parents [96–102]. In a review article on the comorbidity of MDD and ADHD [103] it was concluded, however, that the link between depression and ADHD seemed to be only partially accounted for by comorbid CD or antisocial personality disorder in the family, as depression also was increased in relatives of children with ADHD without CD in some studies. Comorbid MDD and ADHD in children and their first-degree relatives seemed to be influenced by psychosocial risk factors, i.e. marital discord, low social class, large family size, paternal criminality, maternal mental disorder and foster placement, rather than genetic risk factors [104, 105]. Depression in mothers has been related to increased ODD and CD symptoms, predominantely in boys with or without ADHD, therefore presenting a major environmental risk factor for ADHD comorbid with other psychiatric disorders [85, 106].

In addition to MDD, an increased rate of bipolar disorder has been suggested in children with ADHD and their first-degree relatives [107, 108]. A recent study in children with bipolar disorder and ADHD, however, did show that bipolar disorder-I in children and adults share the same diathesis, and ADHD is another, unrelated disorder [109].

A few family studies have explored familiality of ADHD with specific learning disability [110–112]. Specific learning disability and low IQ did not cosegregate with ADHD in most studies despite high rates of reading and writing disability in children with ADHD [113]. These findings differ from the results of twin studies on reading disability and ADHD (see above), which might be due lack of a separate assessment of the inattentive subtype in the family studies.

Other comorbid disorders, which are frequently found to be associated with ADHD in clinical or epidemiological samples, like primary nocturnal enuresis [114] or tic disorders [115, 116], were rarely explored in family studies on ADHD. Two family studies have been performed with regard to ADHD comorbid with Tourette's disorder (TD) [111, 117]. Both studies suggested some relationship of TD with ADHD, however the hypothesis that cases of ADHD might represent a variant expression of TD was refuted. Likewise, TD seemed not to be simply a variant expression of

ADHD. ADHD+TD as well as ADHD and TD seemed to co-occur more frequently in some families, implying heterogeneity in ADHD with regard to comorbid TD. In ADHD+TD families, additionally increased rates of obsessive compulsive disorders (OCD) were found, which also have been described in other studies, implying a unique familial subtype [118, 119].

Longitudinal Family Studies

Three longitudinal family studies have been published which focused on the differences between families of children with ADHD without and with comorbid CD. The first study did follow a sample of 140 children with ADHD and 120 normal control children and their siblings for 4 years into adolescence, who were compared with regard to DSM-III-R diagnoses derived from diagnostic interviews with mother and child. Cross-sectional data did show a higher risk for CD in siblings of children and adolescents with ADHD+CD, but not for children with ADHD+ODD or ADHD alone. This pattern was maintained over the 4-year follow-up period, pointing towards ADHD+CD as a distinct subtype of ADHD [103]. In the second study, a somewhat different approach was taken assessing antisocial families, defined by the presence of antisocial personality disorder in a parent according to DSM-III-R [120]. Antisocial personality disorder in a parent at baseline predicted the presence of CD and ODD in the child 4 years later. Siblings of ADHD children with antisocial personality disorder in a parent compared to families of children without had higher rates of alcohol or drug abuse or dependence. ADHD children from antisocial families did differ from ADHD children from non-antisocial families with regard to comorbid CD and alcohol or drug abuse or dependence, after correcting for IQ differences. Elevated rates of ODD, anxiety disorders and MDD were found in both types of ADHD families. Together with the results of cross-sectional studies [81], the longitudinal studies therefore point towards ADHD+CD as a distinct subtype of ADHD, not including ODD.

Family Studies in Adult Individuals with ADHD

Despite increasing knowledge about ADHD persisting from childhood into adulthood [121] and recognition of adult ADHD [122], family studies on individuals with adult ADHD and their children or other relatives are scarce. Patterns of comorbidities in adults with ADHD are similar to psychiatric disorder patterns found in parents of children with ADHD, i.e. increased rates of comorbid MDD, dysthymia, anxiety disorders, conduct or antisocial personality disorder and substance abuse/dependence with highest rates in the DSM-IV combined ADHD subtype [122–125]. However, from these patterns, no conclusions with regard to specific genetically or environmentally influenced subtypes can be drawn. Studies on the impact of exposure to parental ADHD on their offspring did show an increased risk for ADHD in children of parents with ADHD, also associated with greater environmental risk factors, especially family conflict [126, 127]. Parental ADHD in one study was independent of family conflict, in the other study, family conflict was directly influenced by parental ADHD.

Conclusions

Family and twin studies on ADHD in children and adolescents resulted in a strong heritable component of 60–80% for ADHD. Rates of comorbidity as well as persistence or remittance of the disorder during the lifespan indicate heterogeneity of ADHD, which also might be found regarding the inattentive and the combined ADHD subtype. No clear conclusions can be drawn regarding the pattern of inheritance, as twin and family studies indicate different modes of inheritance, i.e. the oligogenic/polygenic model with additional environmental risk factors for ADHD or a single major gene with low penetrance. Twin and family studies agree with regard to missing sex differences in the genetic risk for ADHD. Similarly, both types of studies pointed towards ADHD+CD as a strongly genetically influenced subtype of ADHD, however also showing some specific environmental risk factors. Another interesting subtype with strong associated genetic risk factors might be persistent ADHD into adulthood. The presented studies did differ considerably with regard to diagnostic criteria, rating scales or interview methods as well as environmental risk factors addressed. Major problems in studies of children and adolescents/adults with ADHD are informant effects with regard to mother/parent and self-rating. Therefore, pervasive ADHD as defined by meeting criteria in two different settings should be used as the target phenotype in molecular genetic studies.

References

1 Willerman L: Activity level and hyperactivity in twins. Child Dev 1973;44:288–293.
2 Goodman R, Stevenson J: A twin study of hyperactivity. II. The aetiological role of genes, family relationships and perinatal adversity. J Child Psychol Psychiatry 1989;30:691–709.
3 Stevenson J: Evidence for a genetic etiology in hyperactivity in children. Behav Genet 1992;22:337–344.
4 Faraone SV, Perlis RH, Doyle AE, et al: Molecular genetics of attention-deficit hyperactivity disorder. Biol Psychiatry 2005;57:1313–1323.
5 Schultz MR, Rabi K, Faraone SV, et al: Efficacy of retrospective recall of attention-deficit hyperactivity disorder symptoms: a twin study. Twin Res Hum Genet 2006;9:220–232.
6 Levy F, Hay DA, McStephen M, et al: Attention-deficit hyperactivity disorder: a category or a continuum? Genetic analysis of a large-scale twin study. J Am Acad Child Adolesc Psychiatry 1997;36:737–744.
7 Sherman DK, McGue MK, Iacono WG: Twin concordance for attention-deficit hyperactivity disorder: a comparison of teachers' and mothers' reports. Am J Psychiatry 1997;154:532–535.
8 Eaves LJ, Silberg JL, Meyer JM, et al: Genetics and developmental psychopathology. 2. The main effects of genes and environment on behavioral problems in the Virginia Twin Study of Adolescent Behavioral Development. J Child Psychol Psychiatry 1997;38:965–980.

9 Nadder TS, Rutter M, Silberg JL, et al: Genetic effects on the variation and covariation of attention-deficit hyperactivity disorder and oppositional-defiant disorder/conduct disorder symptomatologies across informant and occasion of measurement. Psychol Med 2002;32:39–53.
10 Rhee SH, Waldman ID, Hay DA, et al: Sex differences in genetic and environmental influences on DSM-III-R attention-deficit hyperactivity disorder. J Abnorm Psychol 1999;108:24–41.
11 American Psychiatric Association (APA): Diagnostic and Statistical Manual of Mental Disorders. Washington, APA, 1994.
12 Achenbach TM: Manual for the Youth Self Report and 1991 Profile. Burlington, University of Vermont Department of Psychiatry, 1991.
13 Edelbrock C, Rende R, Plomin R, et al: A twin study of competence and problem behavior in childhood and early adolescence. J Child Psychol Psychiatry 1995;36:775–785.
14 Gjone H, Stevenson J, Sundet JM: Genetic influence on parent-reported attention-related problems in a Norwegian general population twin sample. J Am Acad Child Adolesc Psychiatry 1996;35:588–596.
15 Hudziak JJ, Rudiger LP, Neale MC, et al: A twin study of inattentive, aggressive, and anxious/depressed behaviors. J Am Acad Child Adolesc Psychiatry 2000;39:469–476.
16 Rietveld MJ, Hudziak JJ, Bartels M, et al: Heritability of attention problems in children. I. Cross-sectional results from a study of twins, age 3–12 years. Am J Med Genet B Neuropsychiatr Genet 2003;117:102–113.
17 Sherman DK, Iacono WG, McGue MK: Attention-deficit hyperactivity disorder dimensions: a twin study of inattention and impulsivity-hyperactivity. J Am Acad Child Adolesc Psychiatry 1997;36:745–753.
18 Silberg J, Rutter M, Meyer J, et al: Genetic and environmental influences on the covariation between hyperactivity and conduct disturbance in juvenile twins. J Child Psychol Psychiatry 1996;37:803–816.
19 Thapar A, Hervas A, McGuffin P: Childhood hyperactivity scores are highly heritable and show sibling competition effects: twin study evidence. Behav Genet 1995;25:537–544.
20 Nadder TS, Silberg JL, Rutter M, et al: Comparison of multiple measures of ADHD symptomatology: a multivariate genetic analysis. J Child Psychol Psychiatry 2001;42:475–486.
21 Hudziak JJ, Heath AC, Madden PF, et al: Latent class and factor analysis of DSM-IV ADHD: a twin study of female adolescents. J Am Acad Child Adolesc Psychiatry 1998;37:848–857.
22 Neuman RJ, Todd RD, Heath AC, et al: Evaluation of ADHD typology in three contrasting samples: a latent class approach. J Am Acad Child Adolesc Psychiatry 1999;38:25–33.
23 Rasmussen ER, Neuman RJ, Heath AC, et al: Replication of the latent class structure of attention-deficit hyperactivity disorder subtypes in a sample of Australian twins. J Child Psychol Psychiatry 2002;43:1018–1028.
24 Todd RD, Rasmussen ER, Neuman RJ, et al: Familiality and heritability of subtypes of attention-deficit hyperactivity disorder in a population sample of adolescent female twins. Am J Psychiatry 2001; 158:1891–1898.
25 Rasmussen ER, Neuman RJ, Heath AC, et al: Familial clustering of latent class and DSM-IV defined attention-deficit hyperactivity disorder subtypes. J Child Psychol Psychiatry 2004;45:589–598.
26 Simonoff E, Pickles A, Hervas A, et al: Genetic influences on childhood hyperactivity: contrast effects imply parental rating bias, not sibling interaction. Psychol Med 1998;28:825–837.
27 Thapar A, Harrington R, Ross K, et al: Does the definition of ADHD affect heritability? J Am Acad Child Adolesc Psychiatry 2000;39:1528–1536.
28 Martin N, Scourfield J, McGuffin P: Observer effects and heritability of childhood attention-deficit hyperactivity disorder symptoms. Br J Psychiatry 2002;180:260–265.
29 Kuntsi J, Rijsdijk F, Ronald A, et al: Genetic influences on the stability of attention-deficit hyperactivity disorder symptoms from early to middle childhood. Biol Psychiatry 2005;57:647–654.
30 Saudino KJ, Ronald A, Plomin R: The etiology of behavior problems in 7-year-old twins: substantial genetic influence and negligible shared environmental influence for parent ratings and ratings by same and different teachers. J Abnorm Child Psychol 2005;33:113–130.
31 Hay DA, Bennett KS, Levy F, et al: A twin study of attention-deficit hyperactivity disorder dimensions rated by the Strengths and Weaknesses of ADHD-Symptoms and Normal-Behavior (SWAN) scale. Biol Psychiatry 2007;61:700–705.
32 Costello EJ, Loeber R, Stouthamer-Loeber M: Pervasive and situational hyperactivity – confounding effect of informant: a research note. J Child Psychol Psychiatry 1991;32:367–376.
33 Graetz BW, Sawyer MG, Baghurst P: Gender differences among children with DSM-IV ADHD in Australia. J Am Acad Child Adolesc Psychiatry 2005;44:159–168.
34 Willcutt EG, Pennington BF, Chhabildas NA, et al: Psychiatric comorbidity associated with DSM-IV ADHD in a non-referred sample of twins. J Am Acad Child Adolesc Psychiatry 1999;38:1355–1362.

35 Levy F, Hay DA, Bennett KS, et al: Gender differences in ADHD subtype comorbidity. J Am Acad Child Adolesc Psychiatry 2005;44:368–376.
36 Nadder TS, Silberg JL, Eaves LJ, et al: Genetic effects on ADHD symptomatology in 7- to 13-year-old twins: results from a telephone survey. Behav Genet 1998;28:83–99.
37 Rhee SH, Waldman ID: Etiology of sex differences in the prevalence of ADHD: an examination of inattention and hyperactivity-impulsivity. Am J Med Genet B Neuropsychiatr Genet 2004;127:60–64.
38 Offord DR, Boyle MH, Szatmari P, et al: Ontario Child Health Study. II. Six-month prevalence of disorder and rates of service utilization. Arch Gen Psychiatry 1987;44:832–836.
39 Willcutt EG, Pennington BF, DeFries JC: Twin study of the etiology of comorbidity between reading disability and attention-deficit hyperactivity disorder. Am J Med Genet 2000;96:293–301.
40 Friedman MC, Chhabildas N, Budhiraja N, et al: Etiology of the comorbidity between RD and ADHD: exploration of the non-random mating hypothesis. Am J Med Genet B Neuropsychiatr Genet 2003;120:109–115.
41 Gilger JW, Pennington BF, DeFries JC: A twin study of the etiology of comorbidity: attention-deficit hyperactivity disorder and dyslexia. J Am Acad Child Adolesc Psychiatry 1992;31:343–348.
42 Levy F, Hay D, McLaughlin M, et al: Twin sibling differences in parental reports of ADHD, speech, reading and behaviour problems. J Child Psychol Psychiatry 1996;37:569–578.
43 Trzesniewski KH, Moffitt TE, Caspi A, et al: Revisiting the association between reading achievement and antisocial behavior: new evidence of an environmental explanation from a twin study. Child Dev 2006;77:72–88.
44 Thapar A, Harrington R, McGuffin P: Examining the comorbidity of ADHD-related behaviours and conduct problems using a twin study design. Br J Psychiatry 2001;179:224–229.
45 Dick DM, Viken RJ, Kaprio J, et al: Understanding the covariation among childhood externalizing symptoms: genetic and environmental influences on conduct disorder, attention-deficit hyperactivity disorder, and oppositional defiant disorder symptoms. J Abnorm Child Psychol 2005,33:219–229.
46 Burt SA, Krueger RF, McGue M, et al: Sources of covariation among attention-deficit hyperactivity disorder, oppositional defiant disorder, and conduct disorder: the importance of shared environment. J Abnorm Psychol 2001;110:516–525.
47 Burt SA, McGue M, Krueger RF, et al: Sources of covariation among the child-externalizing disorders: informant effects and the shared environment. Psychol Med 2005;35:1133–1144.
48 Barkley RA, Fischer M, Smallish L, et al: The persistence of attention-deficit hyperactivity disorder into young adulthood as a function of reporting source and definition of disorder. J Abnorm Psychol 2002; 111:279–289.
49 Neuman RJ, Heath A, Reich W, et al: Latent class analysis of ADHD and comorbid symptoms in a population sample of adolescent female twins. J Child Psychol Psychiatry 2001;42:933–942.
50 Larsson JO, Larsson H, Lichtenstein P: Genetic and environmental contributions to stability and change of ADHD symptoms between 8 and 13 years of age: a longitudinal twin study. J Am Acad Child Adolesc Psychiatry 2004;43:1267–1275.
51 Price TS, Simonoff E, Asherson P, et al: Continuity and change in preschool ADHD symptoms: longitudinal genetic analysis with contrast effects. Behav Genet 2005;35:121–132.
52 Rietveld MJ, Hudziak JJ, Bartels M, et al: Heritability of attention problems in children: longitudinal results from a study of twins, age 3–12. J Child Psychol Psychiatry 2004;45:577–588.
53 Biederman J, Munir K, Knee D, et al: A family study of patients with attention-deficit disorder and normal controls. J Psychiatr Res 1986;20:263–274.
54 Morrison JR: Childhood hyperactivity in an adult psychiatric population: social factors. J Clin Psychiatry 1980;41:40–43.
55 Asbury K, Dunn JF, Plomin R: Birthweight-discordance and differences in early parenting relate to monozygotic twin differences in behaviour problems and academic achievement at age 7. Dev Sci 2006;9:F22–F31.
56 Lehn H, Derks EM, Hudziak JJ, et al: Attention problems and attention-deficit hyperactivity disorder in discordant and concordant monozygotic twins: evidence of environmental mediators. J Am Acad Child Adolesc Psychiatry 2007;46:83–91.
57 Linnet KM, Wisborg K, Obel C, et al: Smoking during pregnancy and the risk for hyperkinetic disorder in offspring. Pediatrics 2005;116:462–467.
58 Linnet KM, Dalsgaard S, Obel C, et al: Maternal lifestyle factors in pregnancy risk of attention-deficit hyperactivity disorder and associated behaviors: review of the current evidence. Am J Psychiatry 2003;160:1028–1040.
59 Sprich S, Biederman J, Crawford MH, et al: Adoptive and biological families of children and adolescents with ADHD. J Am Acad Child Adolesc Psychiatry 2000;39:1432–1437.
60 Cantwell DP: Genetic studies of hyperactive children: psychiatric illness in biologic and adopting parents. Proc Annu Meet Am Psychopathol Assoc 1975;273–280.

61 Morrison JR, Stewart MA: The psychiatric status of the legal families of adopted hyperactive children. Arch Gen Psychiatry 1973;28:888–891.
62 Alberts-Corush J, Firestone P, Goodman JT: Attention and impulsivity characteristics of the biological and adoptive parents of hyperactive and normal control children. Am J Orthopsychiatry 1986;56:413–423.
63 Maher BS, Marazita ML, Moss HB, et al: Segregation analysis of attention-deficit hyperactivity disorder. Am J Med Genet 1999;88:71–78.
64 Hebebrand J, Dempfle A, Saar K, et al: A genome-wide scan for attention-deficit hyperactivity disorder in 155 German sib-pairs. Mol Psychiatry 2006;11:196–205.
65 August GJ, Stewart MA: Familial subtypes of childhood hyperactivity. J Nerv Ment Dis 1983;171:362–368.
66 Lahey BB, Piacentini JC, McBurnett K, et al: Psychopathology in the parents of children with conduct disorder and hyperactivity. J Am Acad Child Adolesc Psychiatry 1988;27:163–170.
67 Morrison JR, Stewart MA: A family study of the hyperactive child syndrome. Biol Psychiatry 1971;3:189–195.
68 Reeves JC, Werry JS, Elkind GS, et al: Attention-deficit, conduct, oppositional, and anxiety disorders in children. II. Clinical characteristics. J Am Acad Child Adolesc Psychiatry 1987;26:144–155.
69 Stewart MA, DeBlois CS, Cummings C: Psychiatric disorder in the parents of hyperactive boys and those with conduct disorder. J Child Psychol Psychiatry 1980;21:283–292.
70 Stewart MA, Morrison JR: Affective disorder among the relatives of hyperactive children. J Child Psychol Psychiatry 1973;14:209–212.
71 Schachar R, Wachsmuth R: Hyperactivity and parental psychopathology. J Child Psychol Psychiatry 1990;31:381–392.
72 Epstein JN, Conners CK, Erhardt D, et al: Familial aggregation of ADHD characteristics. J Abnorm Child Psychol 2000;28:585–594.
73 Faraone SV, Biederman J, Keenan K, et al: A family-genetic study of girls with DSM-III attention-deficit disorder. Am J Psychiatry 1991;148:112–117.
74 Faraone SV, Biederman J, Milberger S: An exploratory study of ADHD among second-degree relatives of ADHD children. Biol Psychiatry 1994;35:398–402.
75 Faraone SV, Biederman J, Mick E, et al: Family study of girls with attention-deficit hyperactivity disorder. Am J Psychiatry 2000;157:1077–1083.
76 Stawicki JA, Nigg JT, von Eye A: Family psychiatric history evidence on the nosological relations of DSM-IV ADHD combined and inattentive subtypes: new data and meta-analysis. J Child Psychol Psychiatry 2006;47:935–945.
77 Faraone SV, Biederman J, Friedman D: Validity of DSM-IV subtypes of attention-deficit hyperactivity disorder: a family study perspective. J Am Acad Child Adolesc Psychiatry 2000;39:300–307.
78 Smalley SL, McGough JJ, Del'Homme M, et al: Familial clustering of symptoms and disruptive behaviors in multiplex families with attention-deficit hyperactivity disorder. J Am Acad Child Adolesc Psychiatry 2000;39:1135–1143.
79 Faraone SV, Biederman J, Mick E, et al: A family study of psychiatric comorbidity in girls and boys with attention-deficit hyperactivity disorder. Biol Psychiatry 2001;50:586–592.
80 Rhee SH, Waldman ID: Sex differences in genetic and environmental influences on DSM-III-R attention-deficit hyperactivity disorder. J Abnorm Psychol 1999;108:24–41.
81 Faraone SV, Biederman J, Chen WJ, et al: Genetic heterogeneity in attention-deficit hyperactivity disorder: gender, psychiatric comorbidity, and maternal attention-deficit hyperactivity disorder. J Abnorm Psychol 1995;104:334–345.
82 Rhee SH, Hewitt JK, Corley RP, et al: The validity of analyses testing the etiology of comorbidity between two disorders: a review of family studies. J Child Psychol Psychiatry 2003;44:612–636.
83 Faraone SV, Biederman J, Keenan K, et al: Separation of DSM-III attention-deficit disorder and conduct disorder: evidence from a family-genetic study of American child psychiatric patients. Psychol Med 1991;21:109–121.
84 Chronis AM, Lahey BB, Pelham WE Jr, et al: Maternal depression and early positive parenting predict future conduct problems in young children with attention-deficit hyperactivity disorder. Dev Psychol 2007;43:70–82.
85 Chronis AM, Lahey BB, Pelham WE Jr, et al: Psychopathology and substance abuse in parents of young children with attention-deficit hyperactivity disorder. J Am Acad Child Adolesc Psychiatry 2003;42:1424–1432.
86 Faraone SV, Biederman J, Jetton JG, et al: Attention-deficit disorder and conduct disorder: longitudinal evidence for a familial subtype. Psychol Med 1997;27:291–300.
87 Faraone SV, Biederman J, Monuteaux MC: Attention-deficit disorder and conduct disorder in girls: evidence for a familial subtype. Biol Psychiatry 2000;48:21–29.

88 Biederman J, Faraone SV, Keenan K, et al: Family-genetic and psychosocial risk factors in DSM-III attention-deficit disorder. J Am Acad Child Adolesc Psychiatry 1990;29:526–533.
89 Nigg JT, Hinshaw SP: Parent personality traits and psychopathology associated with antisocial behaviors in childhood attention-deficit hyperactivity disorder. J Child Psychol Psychiatry 1998;39:145–159.
90 Biederman J, Faraone SV, Keenan K, et al: Familial association between attention-deficit disorder and anxiety disorders. Am J Psychiatry 1991;148:251–256.
91 Braaten EB, Biederman J, Monuteaux MC, et al: Revisiting the association between attention-deficit hyperactivity disorder and anxiety disorders: a familial risk analysis. Biol Psychiatry 2003;53:93–99.
92 Biederman J, Munir K, Knee D, et al: High rate of affective disorders in probands with attention-deficit disorder and in their relatives: a controlled family study. Am J Psychiatry 1987;144:330–333.
93 Biederman J, Faraone SV, Keenan K, et al: Evidence of familial association between attention-deficit disorder and major affective disorders. Arch Gen Psychiatry 1991;48:633–642.
94 Biederman J, Faraone SV, Keenan K, et al: Further evidence for family-genetic risk factors in attention-deficit hyperactivity disorder. Patterns of comorbidity in probands and relatives psychiatrically and pediatrically referred samples. Arch Gen Psychiatry 1992;49:728–738.
95 Bhatia MS, Nigam VR, Bohra N, et al: Attention-deficit disorder with hyperactivity among paediatric outpatients. J Child Psychol Psychiatry 1991;32:297–306.
96 Beardslee WR, Zuckerman BS, Amaro H, et al: Depression among adolescent mothers: a pilot study. J Dev Behav Pediatr 1988;9:62–65.
97 Grigoroiu-Serbanescu M, Christodorescu D, Magureanu S, et al: Adolescent offspring of endogenous unipolar depressive parents and of normal parents. J Affect Disord 1991;21:185–198.
98 Orvaschel H, Walsh-Allis G, Ye WJ: Psychopathology in children of parents with recurrent depression. J Abnorm Child Psychol 1988;16:17–28.
99 Orvaschel H, Weissman MM, Kidd KK: Children and depression – the children of depressed parents; the childhood of depressed patients; depression in children. J Affect Disord 1980;2:1–16.
100 Nomura Y, Wickramaratne PJ, Warner V, et al: Family discord, parental depression, and psychopathology in offspring: ten-year follow-up. J Am Acad Child Adolesc Psychiatry 2002;41:402–409.
101 Weissman MM, Gammon GD, John K, et al: Children of depressed parents. Increased psychopathology and early onset of major depression. Arch Gen Psychiatry 1987;44:847–853.
102 Weissman MM, Wickramaratne P, Nomura Y, et al: Families at high and low risk for depression: a three-generation study. Arch Gen Psychiatry 2005;62:29–36.
103 Faraone SV, Biederman J: Do attention-deficit hyperactivity disorder and major depression share familial risk factors? J Nerv Ment Dis 1997;185:533–541.
104 Biederman J, Milberger S, Faraone SV, et al: Impact of adversity on functioning and comorbidity in children with attention-deficit hyperactivity disorder. J Am Acad Child Adolesc Psychiatry 1995;34:1495–1503.
105 Biederman J, Faraone SV, Monuteaux MC: Differential effect of environmental adversity by gender: Rutter's index of adversity in a group of boys and girls with and without ADHD. Am J Psychiatry 2002;159:1556–1562.
106 Marmorstein NR, Iacono WG: Major depression and conduct disorder in youth: associations with parental psychopathology and parent-child conflict. J Child Psychol Psychiatry 2004;45:377–386.
107 Biederman J, Faraone S, Mick E, et al: Attention-deficit hyperactivity disorder and juvenile mania: an overlooked comorbidity? J Am Acad Child Adolesc Psychiatry 1996;35:997–1008.
108 Faraone SV, Biederman J, Mennin D, et al: Bipolar and antisocial disorders among relatives of ADHD children: parsing familial subtypes of illness. Am J Med Genet 1998;81:108–116.
109 Geller B, Tillman R, Bolhofner K, et al: Controlled, blindly rated, direct-interview family study of a prepubertal and early-adolescent bipolar I disorder phenotype: morbid risk, age at onset, and comorbidity. Arch Gen Psychiatry 2006;63:1130–1138.
110 Doyle AE, Faraone SV, DuPre EP, et al: Separating attention-deficit hyperactivity disorder and learning disabilities in girls: a familial risk analysis. Am J Psychiatry 2001;158:1666–1672.
111 Faraone SV, Biederman J, Lehman BK, et al: Evidence for the independent familial transmission of attention-deficit hyperactivity disorder and learning disabilities: results from a family genetic study. Am J Psychiatry 1993;150:891–895.
112 Pauls DL, Leckman JF, Cohen DJ: Familial relationship between Gilles de la Tourette's syndrome, attention-deficit disorder, learning disabilities, speech disorders, and stuttering. J Am Acad Child Adolesc Psychiatry 1993;32:1044–1050.
113 Del'Homme M, Kim TS, Loo SK, et al: Familial association and frequency of learning disabilities in ADHD sibling pair families. J Abnorm Child Psychol 2007;35:55–62.

114 Baeyens D, Roeyers H, Vande Walle J, et al: Behavioural problems and attention-deficit hyperactivity disorder in children with enuresis: a literature review. Eur J Pediatr 2005;164:665–672.
115 Kadesjo B, Gillberg C: Tourette's disorder: epidemiology and comorbidity in primary schoolchildren. J Am Acad Child Adolesc Psychiatry 2000;39:548–555.
116 Spencer T, Biederman M, Coffey B, et al: The 4-year course of tic disorders in boys with attention-deficit hyperactivity disorder. Arch Gen Psychiatry 1999;56:842–847.
117 Stewart SE, Illmann C, Geller DA, et al: A controlled family study of attention-deficit hyperactivity disorder and Tourette's disorder. J Am Acad Child Adolesc Psychiatry 2006;45:1354–1362.
118 Geller D, Petty C, Vivas F, et al: Examining the relationship between obsessive-compulsive disorder and attention-deficit hyperactivity disorder in children and adolescents: a familial risk analysis. Biol Psychiatry 2007;61:316–321.
119 Spencer T, Biederman J, Harding M, et al: Disentangling the overlap between Tourette's disorder and ADHD. J Child Psychol Psychiatry 1998;39:1037–1044.
120 Faraone SV, Biederman J, Mennin D, et al: Familial subtypes of attention-deficit hyperactivity disorder: a 4-year follow-up study of children from antisocial-ADHD families. J Child Psychol Psychiatry 1998;39:1045–1053.
121 Mannuzza S, Klein RG, Moulton JL 3rd: Persistence of attention-deficit hyperactivity disorder into adulthood: what have we learned from the prospective follow-up studies? J Atten Disord 2003;7:93–100.
122 McGough JJ, Smalley SL, McCracken JT, et al: Psychiatric comorbidity in adult attention-deficit hyperactivity disorder: findings from multiplex families. Am J Psychiatry 2005;162:1621–1627.
123 Biederman J, Faraone SV, Spencer T, et al: Patterns of psychiatric comorbidity, cognition, and psychosocial functioning in adults with attention-deficit hyperactivity disorder. Am J Psychiatry 1993;150:1792–1798.
124 Kessler RC, Adler LA, Barkley R, et al: Patterns and predictors of attention-deficit hyperactivity disorder persistence into adulthood: results from the national comorbidity survey replication. Biol Psychiatry 2005;57:1442–1451.
125 Murphy KR, Barkley RA, Bush T: Young adults with attention-deficit hyperactivity disorder: subtype differences in comorbidity, educational, and clinical history. J Nerv Ment Dis 2002;190:147–157.
126 Biederman J, Faraone SV, Monuteaux MC: Impact of exposure to parental attention-deficit hyperactivity disorder on clinical features and dysfunction in the offspring. Psychol Med 2002;32:817–827.
127 Pressman LJ, Loo SK, Carpenter EM, et al: Relationship of family environment and parental psychiatric diagnosis to impairment in ADHD. J Am Acad Child Adolesc Psychiatry 2006;45:346–354.

Prof. Christine Margarete Freitag, MD, MA
Director, Department of Child and Adolescent Psychiatry
J.W. Goethe-University, Deutschordenstrasse 50
DE–60528 Frankfurt am Main (Germany)
E-Mail c.freitag@em.uni-frankfurt.de

Retz W, Klein RG (eds): Attention-Deficit Hyperactivity Disorder (ADHD) in Adults.
Key Issues in Mental Health. Basel, Karger, 2010, vol 176, pp 58–77

Molecular Genetics of Attention-Deficit Hyperactivity Disorder

Wolfgang Retz[a] · Christine Margarete Freitag[b]

[a]Saarland University Hospital, Institute for Forensic Psychology and Psychiatry, Homburg/Saar, and [b]Department of Child and Adolescent Psychiatry, Frankfurt University Hospital, Frankfurt, Germany

Abstract

Family, twin, and adoption studies support the notion that attention-deficit hyperactivity disorder (ADHD) is a highly heritable disorder. Following from these quantitative genetic findings, numerous molecular genetic associations and a few linkage studies have been performed during the last years. Due to evidence from pharmacological, neuroimaging and animal studies, the majority of the candidate genes studied have focused on various facets of the dopamine, norepinephrine, and serotonin neurotransmitter systems. Meta-analyses and pooled data analyses have supported associations between ADHD and polymorphisms in genes coding for the dopamine D4 and D5 receptors and the dopamine and serotonin transporters, respectively. Linkage analyses give some additional support for an involvement of the dopamine transporter (DAT1) gene in ADHD. Recent studies have started to implicate environmental factors and comorbidity as well as endophenotypes of ADHD in molecular genetic research in order to further elucidate the neurobiological basis of this disorder.

Attention-deficit hyperactivity disorder (ADHD) is a common psychiatric condition usually manifesting itself in childhood with a prevalence of 6–9% in school-age children [1]. Follow-up studies reported persistence of symptoms into adulthood in about 50–60% of affected children. Adults may show either residual symptoms or the full clinical disorder [2–4]. ADHD thus displays all characteristics of a chronic disease. According to current epidemiological studies, the transnational prevalence of adult ADHD is approximately 3.4% on average [5]. Based on these prevalence rates, ADHD probably represents one of the most common mental conditions in adults. ADHD is not limited to a specific social class and does not depend on the level of education [1]. In epidemiological samples, male patients outnumber females by a ratio of 2–3:1 in childhood. In adults the gender ratio tends to be more equal.

Heritability of ADHD has been widely studied in family, twin and adoption studies in children, but rarely in adults [see Freitag and Retz, chapter 2]. Meta-analytic evaluation of 20 twin studies from European states, North America and Australia revealed a mean heritability estimate of 70–80% suggesting that ADHD is among the most heritable of psychiatric disorders [6]. As a common, complex behavioral disorder, the most likely mode of transmission is oligo- or polygenic with some environmental effects contributing to the disorder. This model postulates interactive or epistatic effects of many different genes on different chromosomes, each gene contributing to only a small part of phenotypic variance, and additional interaction with environmental factors [7].

As for any formal and molecular genetic investigation, defining the phenotype is of crucial importance. In all periods of life, i.e. childhood, adolescence and adulthood, the key symptoms and signs of ADHD consist of inattention, hyperactivity and impulsivity. Regarding ADHD, the concepts behind, the criteria for, and the terms of this syndrome have changed frequently. This issue has to be considered in the interpretation of genetic studies in ADHD and complicates a direct comparison of studies in this field. Currently, two diagnostic concepts are used for childhood and adult ADHD, based on the presentation of typical behavioral phenomena, which have been validated in ADHD children and adolescents: DSM-IV-TR [8] and ICD-10 [9]. The validity for the diagnostic criteria used for adult patients by these classifications is under discussion [see Stieglitz, chapter 6]. Although the sets of diagnostic criteria used by DSM-IV-TR and the research version of the international classification of diseases (ICD-10) are nearly identical, there are some substantial differences between 'hyperkinetic disorders' according to ICD-10 and ADHD according to DSM-IV-TR. While the diagnosis of 'hyperkinetic disorder' requires at least 6 symptoms of inattention, 3 symptoms of hyperactivity, and 1 of impulsivity, 'ADHD' according to DSM-IV-TR is diagnosed when at least 6 symptoms of inattention and/or hyperactivity/impulsivity are present. Thus, ICD-10 defines a more severe type of the disorder compared to ADHD-combined type and does not give criteria to diagnose the ADHD-inattentive and ADHD-hyperactive/impulsive subtypes (table 1).

From a genetic point of view, the clinical subtypes of ADHD according to DSM-IV-TR are a matter of debate. A separate analysis of inattention and hyperactivity and impulsivity might be recommendable as some studies were indicative of a different genetic determination of inattention and hyperactivity/impulsivity, however, with some genetic overlap between symptoms. It should be also kept in mind that ADHD is the extreme end of a syndromal dimension, although it is a categorical diagnosis according to DSM-IV-TR and ICD-10, respectively. The diagnostic manuals account for the dimensional character of ADHD by requiring a threshold number of symptoms of inattentiveness and/or hyperactive/impulsive behavior. Although many studies have investigated ADHD as a category, its conceptualization as a quantitative, dimensional trait has been widely used in formal and, to a lesser extent, molecular genetic studies of ADHD. Both the categorical diagnosis or the continuously distributed trait approach are feasible for molecular genetic studies, as definition of ADHD by continuous or categorical data does not change the

Table 1. Diagnosis of ADHD according to ICD-10 and DSM-IV-TR

Diagnosis	Number of criteria needed			Conduct disorder
	inattention	hyperactivity	impulsivity	
DSM-IV				
ADHD combined type	≥6/9	≥6/9		comorbid
ADHD inattentive type	≥6/9	<6/9		diagnosis
ADHD hyperactive/impulsive type	<6/9	≥6/9		if applicable
ICD-10				
Hyperkinetic disorder	≥6/9	≥3/5	≥1/4	no
Hyperkinetic disorder of conduct	≥6/9	≥3/5	≥1/4	yes

resulting estimates of an additive genetic effect in the range of 75–90% [see Freitag and Retz, chapter 2].

Another problem that has to be considered in genetic studies concerns the source of information that might influence phenotype description. In adults, diagnosis of ADHD primarily relies on symptom description by the patient. Up to now it is not clear whether the possibility to explore psychopathological symptoms in adults and the development of special sets of diagnostic criteria, like the Utah criteria [see Wender and Tomb, chapter 1], will help to refine the ADHD phenotype.

Comorbidity with other psychiatric disorders is a widely recognized phenomenon, which has been confirmed in a large number of studies [see Klein and Mannuzza, chapter 7]. The nature of relationship of ADHD and comorbid disorders is not well understood, but the high coincidence rates of genetically determined complex disorders suggest the presence of neurobiological links. Although DSM-IV-TR requires a separate classification of psychiatric disorders co-occurring with ADHD, comorbidity of psychopathological syndromes with ADHD might represent not only clinical ADHD subtypes, but clinically distinct disorders, caused by infrequent mutations in a small number of patients. It could be shown that conduct disorder but not anxiety and affective disorders co-segregate within ADHD families [10] and it has been concluded from a series of family studies that ADHD with conduct disorder is genetically distinct from pure ADHD [11, 12]. On the other hand it has been argued that polygenic inheritance of ADHD might explain the high comorbidity rates with other complex and likely polygenetic comorbid disorders. Due to this model, ADHD shares a number of common, pleiotropic genes with other disorders, for example conduct disorder. Given heterogeneity in ADHD, future genetic studies should improve phenotyping of subjects by assessment of comorbidity. Another possibility to overcome this difficulty in ADHD research is the use of endophenotypes, e.g. in terms of neuropsychological assessments or neurophysiologic measures [see Baehne and Fallgatter, chapter 4], which are closer to the biological substrate than the behavioral phenotype.

Linkage Analyses

Genomewide scans offer an important approach to search for genetic risk factors. In contrast to association studies, susceptibility loci can be described without a priori hypotheses on candidate genes. Several independent groups have performed genomewide scans of ADHD [13–23] using sib-pair and multigenerational pedigree approaches. The reports of Smalley et al. [14] and Ogdie et al. [17] are based on an extended sample of the Fisher et al. [13] study. The results shown in table 2 are not unequivocal and might be explained by unavoidable stochastic fluctuations due to the limited sample sizes, or might be due to genetic and clinical heterogeneity of the samples. Given that the method of linkage analysis is known to have low power for genes of small effect and that ADHD is a polygenetic and heterogenetic disorder, the variable pattern of linkage results are no surprise. However, although the studies performed so far did not reveal identical results, the results coincide to some respect. Some chromosome regions such as 5p13, 14q12, and 17p11 have been indicated in multiple studies. First of all, linkage to chromosome 5p has been reported by almost all studies, however the reported lod scores did not exceed significant thresholds in all samples. This finding is of special interest because the dopamine transporter (DAT1) gene is located on this chromosome and dopaminergic pathways are supposed to play a key role in ADHD. An association between ADHD and the DAT1 gene has been repeatedly demonstrated and has been shown to contribute to the linkage signal on chromosome 5 in a German linkage study [24]. In addition to linkage to chromosome 5p, other genes that map on the identified loci include several dopaminergic genes (dopamine receptor D1/DRD1 on 5q, dopamine receptor D2/DRD2 on 11q, dopamine decarboxylase/DDC on 7p, dopamine β-hydroxylase/DBH on 9q) and other glutamatergic and cholinergic candidate genes (GRIN2a on 16p, CHRNA7 on 15q). The concordance between results from different analytical methods of linkage and the replication of data between independent studies suggest that some of the loci identified might truly harbor ADHD susceptibility genes. Interestingly, some of these loci have been suggested to be linked to other developmental neuropsychiatric disorders which share psychopathological symptoms with ADHD, like chromosome 16p and autism.

In order to provide more power to detect true linkage signals, a combined analysis of seven previous studies was performed by the genome scan meta-analysis method [25]. This analysis revealed the most significant linkage to chromosome region from 16q23.1 to the q terminal, which has been identified also in earlier studies, at least on a nominal level [16, 17, 21, 22]. Even in studies which found no linkage signal in this chromosome region, the ranks of these regions were higher than average [15, 19, 20]. Nine additional regions on chromosomes 5, 6, 7, 8, 9, 15, 16, and 17 showed nominal or suggestive linkage signals, which might focus further research on novel susceptibility genes.

Table 2. Linkage analyses in ADHD samples

Reference (first author)	Subjects	Chromosome	Lod scores (>1)
Fisher 2002 [13]	126 affected sib pairs USA	5p12	1.05
		9q22	1.38
		10q26	1.66
		11q25	1.07
		12q23	1.54
		12q24	1.09
		13q12	1.13
		16p13	1.51
		Xp22	1.03
Smalley 2002 [14]	277 affected sib pairs USA	16p13	4.20
Ogdie et al. 2003 [17] 2004 [18]	270 affected sib pairs The Netherlands	5p13	2.55
		6q12	3.30
		11q25	1.27
		16p13	3.73
		17p11	3.63
		20q13	1.19
Bakker 2003 [16]	164 affected sib pairs The Netherlands	3q13.32	1.36
		4p16.3	1.78
		5p13.1	1.43
		6q26	1.19
		7p13	3.04
		9q33.3	2.05
		10cen	1.26
		13q33.3	1.91
		15q15.1	3.54
Arcos-Burgos 2004 [15]	16 multigenerational families Columbia	5q33.3	1.07
		11q22	1.09
		17p11	1.42
Hebebrand 2006 [19]	155 affected sib pairs Germany	5p	2.59
		8	1.29
		12q	2.10
		17p	1.39
Asherson 2008 [21]	142 affected sib pairs Europe	2	1.64
		9q22	2.13
		11	1.31
		14	1.75
		16q23	3.10
		21	1.53
		X	1.25

Table 2. Continued

Reference (first author)	Subjects	Chromosome	Lod scores (>1)
Romanos 2008 [22]	8 multigenerational families Germany	2q35	3.40
		5q13.1	4.16
		6q22-23	3.32
		7q21.11	3.14
		9q22	3.30
		14q12	4.50
		16q24.1	3.26
Faraone 2008 [20]	217 families with 601 affected siblings USA	–	–
Amin 2009 [23]	1 multigenerational family The Netherlands	6p22	1.67
		18q21-22	1.83

Association Studies

Association studies in ADHD were started more than 10 years ago and their number is still growing rapidly. Most studies have been performed in samples of children and adolescents. The majority of studies assessing susceptibility genes for ADHD have focused on molecules which are involved in the regulation of monoaminergic neurotransmission. Other transmitter systems (cholinergic, glutamatergic) have been investigated to a much lesser extent. Despite the problem of population stratification in association studies, the approach has been very fruitful for ADHD research [for detailed reviews also see 6, 26–28]. Inconsistencies between association studies are not unusual and may reflect variation in subject ascertainment and phenotype definition (e.g. quantitative/dimensional vs. qualitative/categorical, with or without comorbidities), differences in ethnicity, differing allele frequencies between populations, genetic heterogeneity, epigenetic diversity, different study designs (family-based vs. case-control) or low statistical power to detect small effects of single genes. Nevertheless, some of the results have been found to be quite robust. The following section intends to give an overview about those findings, which were replicated and confirmed in pooled or meta-analyses.

Dopamine Transporter Gene

Dopaminergic neurotransmission has been supposed to play a key role in ADHD. Given that methylphenidate is known to work by inhibition of the dopamine transporter, the DAT1 gene is a suitable candidate for genetic ADHD research. Moreover, DAT1 knockout mice exhibit features of hyperactivity, which can be reduced by methylphenidate application [29]. Additionally, it has been shown in single photon emission computed tomography studies on adult ADHD subjects that dopamine transporter availability [30] and binding potential [31] differs as a function of DAT1 genotype. In addition, increased density of dopamine transporter in ADHD [32, 33] and normalization with methylphenidate administration have been reported [33].

A finding that has been widely investigated and reported is the association between the 10-repeat allele of a 40-basepair (bp) VNTR in exon 15 of the DAT1 gene. Initially reported by Cook et al. [34], an overrepresentation of the 10-repeat allele in ADHD subjects was replicated in a number of studies all over the world. Association of the DAT1 locus with ADHD was also confirmed in multimarker haplotype analyses [35, 36]. These studies showed evidence for an association between ADHD and DAT1 haplotypes, which also included the 10-repeat allele. However, a number of published studies failed to replicate this finding [37–39].

In an attempt to clarify this inconsistency, all published studies until October 2005 in European and Asian populations were evaluated by a meta-analysis [40]. In this analysis, no compelling evidence for association with the 10-repeat allele of DAT (OR 1.04, 95% CI 0.98–1.11) was found. A similar finding was reported by Maher et al. [41], who analyzed combined data from 11 family-based samples (OR 1.27, 95% CI 0.99–1.63). In contrast, Curran et al. [42] found a small but significant association (OR 1.16), when datasets from nine studies were pooled. Faraone et al. [6] reported an OR of 1.13 (95% CI 1.03–1.24) in family-based studies, suggesting that the dopamine transporter gene merits further investigation but that its effect is modest. Interestingly, in the German genome-scan sample [19] no association between ADHD and the DAT1 10-repeat allele was found, although linkage to the locus that harbors DAT1 was high. It was argued that the reported association between ADHD and the DAT1 10-repeat allele might be mediated by genes which are in linkage disequilibrium. Meanwhile, fine mapping of the DAT1 locus on chromosome 5p13 supports this consideration [24].

Pharmacogenetic studies concerning efficacy of stimulants in the treatment of ADHD have focused on the function of the dopaminergic system and the DAT1 gene in particular. In an Irish sample, an association between the DAT1 10-repeat allele and response to methylphenidate was demonstrated by Kirley et al. [43]. Similarly, Joober et al. [44] reported a better response to methylphenidate in carriers of at least one DAT1 10-repeat allele compared to individuals homozygous to the 9-repeat allele. Children with the 9/9 genotype displayed a distinct dose-response curve without linear symptom improvement with increased methylphenidate doses [45]. In contrast, no influence of this polymorphism with response to methylphenidate treatment was found in other studies [46, 47].

A possible influence of the DAT1 VNTR polymorphism on the long-term outcome of ADHD was investigated in the Milwaukee Longitudinal Study population. In this study, individuals heterozygous for the 9- and 10-repeat allele differed from individuals homozygous for the 10-repeat allele in many respects, suggesting the heterozygous 9/10 genotype or a linked locus to be associated with more ADHD symptoms and externalizing behavior from childhood to adulthood, and therefore also with increased family, educational, and occupational impairments [48].

Dopamine Receptor Genes

Association studies have focused on a number of dopaminergic genes in addition to DAT1, including dopamine receptors D1–5 genes (DRD1, DRD2, DRD3, DRD4, DRD5), the dopamine β-hydroxylase (DBH) gene and the dopamine decarboxylase (DDC) gene. Findings of an association of a 48-bp variable number of tandem repeat polymorphism in exon 3 of the DRD4 gene with 'novelty seeking' [49] have stimulated a large number of association studies in ADHD patients. Moreover, DRD4 mRNA is found predominately in frontal and prefrontal brain regions, and the VNTR polymorphism has been shown to be associated with prefrontal gray matter reduction [50]. The initial finding of an association between ADHD and the DRD4 7-repeat allele [51] has been replicated in several studies by independent research groups. Nevertheless, negative findings also have been reported repeatedly. Positive association might particularly depend on conduct problems comorbid with ADHD [52]. Gornick et al. [53] recently reported an association of the 7-repeat allele with better cognitive performance and favorable long-term outcome within the ADHD patient group in a follow-up study. According to this finding, more externalizing and internalizing behavior was found in 6-year-old children lacking the DRD4 7-repeat allele [54].

While the vast majority of association studies have focused on the DRD4 VNTR polymorphism in exon 3, there are additional studies which reported associations of several polymorphisms and haplotypes of the DRD4 gene [55–57].

In a meta-analysis on the original data and 22 further studies, a small but significant association of the DRD4 7-repeat allele was found with a combined odds ratio of 1.9 (95% CI 1.5–2.2) in case-control studies and 1.4 (95% CI 1.1–1.6) in family-based studies [58]. This meta-analysis aimed to avoid publication bias by using the method of Egger et al. [59]. Of 8 case-control studies, 5 showed a significant association, but only 2 of 14 family-based studies. A second meta-analysis of DRD4, which included data from 13 studies with a total of 571 informative meioses, confirmed these results. The pooled odds ratio estimate was 1.41 (95% CI 1.20–1.64), demonstrating positive association [41]. There was no support of heterogeneity between the included studies. Li et al. [40] recently published a third meta-analysis of all published studies of European and Asian populations until October 2005 to give a comprehensive picture of the role of the DRD4 VNTR polymorphism. They found an OR of 1.34 (95% CI 1.23–1.45), demonstrating a positive association of the DRD4 7-repeat allele.

Replicated associations confirmed by meta-analyses have been also reported for the DRD5 gene. In 1999, Daly et al. [60] reported a significant association between ADHD and the 148-bp allele of a microsatellite marker located 18.5 kb 5′ to the DRD5 gene on chromosome 4. The joint analysis of 14 independent samples showed association of the common 148-bp allele with ADHD (OR 1.24, 95% CI 1.12–1.38) [61]. Also the meta-analysis of Li et al. [40] revealed an increased risk for ADHD conferred by DRD5 148-bp allele (OR 1.34, 95% CI 1.21–1.49), whereas the DRD5 136-bp allele showed protective effects (OR 0.57, 95% CI 0.34–0.96). A positive OR of 1.57 (95% CI 1.25–1.96) was also calculated by Maher et al. [41], who combined samples from 5 studies in their analysis.

The other dopamine receptor subtype genes (DRD1–3) have been less extensively studied in ADHD than DRD4 and DRD5. So far, there is no compelling evidence for involvement of these genes in ADHD etiopathology.

Dopamine-Catalyzing Enzymes

Dopamine β-hydroxylase (DBH) has been considered as candidate gene in ADHD because of its function in degrading dopamine to norepinephrine. Most association studies of the DBH gene with ADHD have focused on a single nucleotide polymorphism, commonly known as DBH TaqI A. Association of this polymorphism with plasma DBH activity has been demonstrated [62]. Moreover, association with the A2 allele of a TaqI polymorphism in intron 5 of the DBH gene in an Irish sample has been reported by Daly et al. [60]. In an extended study using the same sample and several additional markers, haplotypes in this gene were investigated, but only one haplotype (including the TaqI polymorphism) showed significant association with ADHD [36]. The positive association of the TaqI A2 allele was replicated in a Brazilian sample [63]. Wigg et al. [64] found only a trend for a preferential transmission of the TaqI A2 allele in a Canadian ADHD population. Other attempts to replicate this association failed [65, 66]. In the Milwaukee Longitudinal Study sample, TaqI A2 homozygosity was associated with more hyperactivity in childhood, more pervasive behavior problems at adolescence and poorer performance on a neuropsychological task in adulthood [48]. In conclusion, there is some evidence that the DBH gene may confer increased susceptibility towards ADHD, but clarification is needed in further replication studies with independent samples.

Candidate genes, which have been also investigated in ADHD, comprise dopamine decarboxylase, catechol-O-methyltransferase, monoaminooxidase A and B and tyrosine hydroxylase. Although some positive results have been reported, replication has been difficult and results are not unequivocal. Further investigations are needed to rule out false-positive findings and to confirm real associations [6, 26, 28].

Noradrenergic Genes

Dysfunctional noradrenergic neurotransmission has been supposed to contribute to ADHD, based on its important role in the maintenance of attention and vigilance. The norepinephrine transporter (NET1) plays an important role for norepinephrine and dopamine degradation in frontal cortex. Consistent with this hypothesis, atomoxetine, an effective medication for ADHD, is a selective noradrenergic reuptake inhibitor. Several polymorphisms have been identified in coding and non-coding regions of the NET1 gene and were investigated in ADHD samples. The first studies did not support the NET1 gene as a genetic susceptibility factor in ADHD [67–69]. In a more recent study, however, Bobb et al. [70] reported a significant association of two NET1 single nucleotide polymorphisms in family-based, but not in case-control analyses. In the same year, another study [71] identified three NET1 SNPs which showed suggestive association with ADHD, but none of these were significant after adjustment for the number of markers analyzed. Interestingly, two of the three SNPs were those reported by Bobb et al. [70]. Kim et al. [72] found an association of ADHD with a common functional single nucleotide polymorphism (A3081T) in the NET1 promoter region. This result gives further evidence that the NET1 gene might modulate the risk for ADHD. In addition, another NET1 SNP (G1287A) did influence therapeutic response in a small group of children treated with methylphenidate [73]. Therefore, NET1 remains an interesting candidate for further association studies in ADHD.

Concerning noradrenergic receptors, α1c (ADRA1c), α2a (ADRA2), and α2c (ADRA2c) receptor genes have been examined in ADHD samples. Although some associations with polymorphisms within these genes were found, replication has been difficult and some studies reported conflicting results [74–78].

Serotonergic Genes

Interest in the serotonergic system in ADHD has been fuelled by animal studies, showing that methylphenidate decreases hyperlocomotion in DAT1 knockout mice via serotonergic mechanisms [29]. Moreover, the well-established association of low serotonin (5-HT) activity with high impulsiveness made the serotonergic system one of the most extensive studied transmitter systems in ADHD [79].

A 44-bp insertion/depletion polymorphism in the promotor region of the 5-HT transporter gene (5-HTTLPR) has been investigated in a number of studies. Seeger et al. [80] reported an overrepresentation of the long allele variant (L) in hyperkinetic children, which was more pronounced in subjects without comorbid conduct disorder. Corresponding to this finding, Retz et al. [81] observed an association of the 5-HTTLPR L-allele with a dimensional measure of ADHD symptoms in a population of socially maladapted males. Similarly, Manor et al. [82] and Zoroglu et al. [83] found a lower frequency of the short allele (S) in ADHD children. In another case-control study, aggressive children with ADHD were more likely to have at least one 5-HTTLPR L-allele compared to controls [84]. In an analysis of pooled data, which included their own sample and those investigated by Seeger et al. [80] and Manor et al. [82], Kent et al. [85] observed a significant association of ADHD with the 5-HTTLPR L-allele, although they found no association in their sample when analyzed separately. Using a dimensional approach, Curran et al. [86] found further evidence for an association of increased ADHD symptoms with the 5-HTTLPR L-allele and five further markers spanning this region, but not for the VNTR in intron 2 and the 3′UTR SNP. Another study, again, did not find an association with the VNTR in intron 2 with ADHD, but reported preferential transmission of the 5-HTTLPR S-allele, and a haplotype including the VNTR in intron 2 and the 5-HTTLPR L-allele in an Asian sample [87], which appears contradictory. Furthermore, in a regression model including sex and biologic parent status, a significant effect of the 5-HTTLPR on 'externalizing' behaviors including ADHD, conduct disorder and aggressivity has been identified [88]. Kim et al. [89] also failed to identify an association of 5-HTTLPR and VNTR in intron 2 with categorical ADHD. However, further analysis on quantitative measures revealed a positive association with these polymorphisms. In a pooled analysis of European and Asian samples, Xu et al. [90] reported no evidence for association with one of three investigated polymorphisms within the serotonin transporter gene, but significant overrepresentation of a rare haplotype, including the 5-HTTLPR L-allele. No associations with polymorphisms spanning the serotonin transporter gene have been reported in several other studies [91–94]. However, according to the meta-analysis by Faraone et al. [6], the pooled OR for the long allele is 1.31 (95% CI 1.09–1.59), suggesting small but significant effects of the 5-HTTLPR L-allele on ADHD symptoms despite the existing inconsistencies of study results.

Positive association of ADHD with a SNP (G861C) in an untranslated region of the serotonin receptor gene 1b (HTR1b) gene has been reported in two family-based studies. Faraone et al. [6] reported a pooled OR of 1.44 (95% CI 1.14–1.83). Association studies of the serotonin transporter 2a (HTR2a) showed conflicting results. Zoroglu et al. [95] reported no association of ADHD with two SNPs within the HTR2a gene, whereas Levitan et al. [77] found an association with a dimensional measure of ADHD with the C-allele of one of these SNPs (T102C) in a sample of women with seasonal affective disorder. Quist et al. [96] reported no association with the T102C SNP, but a positive association regarding another 5HTR2a polymorphism (His452Tyr), which was not confirmed in a later study, which included four independent samples [97]. However, in one of the four samples, when analyzed alone, preferential transmission of the His allele was reported.

Tryptophan hydroxylase-2 (TPH2) is the rate-limiting enzyme of serotonin synthesis in the brain. Preferential transmission of two SNPs within the regulatory region of this gene (G703T and T473A) has been observed in a German sample [98]. In an Irish sample, overrepresentation of three other SNPs within intron 5 and several haplotypes was associated with ADHD [99]. Brookes et al. [100] also found association with two of these markers, but the risk alleles were opposite to those described by Sheehan et al. [99]. In a second study in a UK sample, Sheehan et al. [101] failed to replicate their first report.

Genomewide Association Studies

Recently, a new generation of association studies has started, which combine the power to detect genetic variants of small sizes, like the 'classical' association studies, with the possibility to perform hypothesis-free analyses of the whole genome, like linkage analyses. These first genomewide association studies (GWAs), which are based either on a sample of 985 parent-child trios from the International Multicentre ADHD Genetics (IMAGE) project [102, 103] or a German sample of 343 ADHD children and adults and 304 controls [104], did not report any associations, which remained formally significant after correction for multiple testing. Interestingly, these GWAs did not support an outstanding role of genes regulating neurotransmission with possible exceptions of a sodium hydrogen carrier gene (SLC9A9), the NOS1 gene, which codes for nitrogen oxidase and the cannabinoid receptor gene (CNR1). However, converging evidence from the two GWAs approaches and also from linkage analyses including the meta-analysis of Zhou et al. [25] provide support for common effects of CDH13 within the chromosomal region 16q23.1-24.3, which codes for T-cadherin, a member of a family of cell-cell adhesion proteins. Although not genomewide significant, the findings of GWA studies point to a minor involvement of genes regulating neurotransmission, but some suggestions are found for involvement of genes coding for cell-cell communication in terms of the regulation of cell adhesion and synaptic plasticity.

Gene-Environment Interactions

Although ADHD is highly heritable, environmental conditions play an important role for its manifestation during childhood development. Besides genetic risk factors, twin studies additionally suggest some influence of shared and non-shared environmental risk factors in ADHD [105]. The most consistent of these are in utero exposure to maternal smoking [106] and low birth weight [107]. Several longitudinal epidemiologic studies assessed psychosocial risk factors including family conflict, child maltreatment, social class, family size, maternal psychopathology, and paternal criminality as risk factors for child psychopathology [108–110]. Recent studies confirmed these risk factors particularly for ADHD [111].

Although neither environmental nor genetic risk factors alone can sufficiently explain ADHD, and possible interactions between both aspects are supposed to be relevant in complex disorders, studies regarding gene by environment interactions in ADHD are rare. Khan et al. [112] reported that the DAT1 10-repeat allele was associated with hyperactive-impulsive symptoms only in those children who were exposed to maternal smoking in utero. A significant interaction between DAT1 genotype and prenatal smoke exposure was also found in another study, indicating that males but not females with prenatal smoke exposure who are homozygous for the DAT1 10-repeat allele have increased measures of hyperactivity-impulsivity [113]. Results of an own investigation suggest that the 5-HTTLPR-mediated risk for ADHD is moderated by environmental adversity and that the impact of environment depends on an individual's genetic background [114]. Analysis of this gene by environment interaction showed that the rate of childhood ADHD in carriers of the LL-genotype was only slightly increased in high compared to low adverse childhood environment risk. With regard to carriers of the SS or SL genotype, a high childhood adverse environment index strongly increased the risk for ADHD in childhood compared to low environment risk. Similarly, a moderating effect of the 5-HTTLPR genotype on environmental effects in ADHD was also found in a recently published study [115].

Conclusions

Formal and molecular genetic studies emphasize the strong role of genetic factors in the etiology of ADHD. Based on results of animal studies and knowledge about the effective pharmacological agents, association studies confirmed the role of genetic variants in genes relevant for monoaminergic neurotransmission in ADHD. In turn, these studies provide neurobiological evidence that ADHD is a valid diagnosis.

Linkage analyses offer an important approach to elicit new chromosomal regions, which might harbor genetic risk factors for ADHD, and are supportive in identifying new susceptibility genes by positional cloning. Whole-genome scans resulted in as yet inconclusive findings with regard to the genetic basis of ADHD and only partially have been supportive of the association studies results. It should be considered in this context that ADHD is a heterogeneous, polygenetic disorder and that all associated genetic variants show only small effects on ADHD symptoms. Furthermore, psychiatric comorbidities and environmental factors might contribute to the phenotypic expression. Thus, there seems to be a need to consider these factors in future linkage analyses and association studies, which also implies the need for much larger sample sizes than used in the studies generated so far. In addition, endophenotypes of ADHD offer an attractive tool for molecular genetic studies, since they might be closer related to the neurobiological substrate of ADHD than behavioral measures and might, therefore, help to bridge the gap between genes and diagnosis.

References

1 Barkley RA, Murphy KR: Attention-Deficit Hyperactivity Disorder. A Clinical Workbook. New York, Guilford Publications, 1998.

2 Weiss G, Hechtman LT, Milroy T, Perlman: Psychiatric status of hyperactives as adults: a controlled prospective 15-year follow-up of 63 hyperactive children. J Am Acad Child Psychiatry 1985;24: 211–220.

3 Mannuzza S, Klein RG, Bessler A, Malloy P, LaPadula M: Adult outcome of hyperactive boys: educational achievement, occupational rank, and psychiatric status. Arch Gen Psychiatry 1993;50:565–576.

4 Barkley RA: Major life activity and health outcomes associated with attention-deficit hyperactivity disorder. J Clin Psychiatry 2002;63(suppl 12):10–15.

5 Fayyad J, De Graaf R, Kessler R, Alonso J, Angermeyer M, Demyttenaere K, De Girolamo G, Haro JM, Karam EG, Lara C, Lépine JP, Ormel J, Posada-Villa J, Zaslavsky AM, Jin R: Cross-national prevalence and correlates of adult attention-deficit hyperactivity disorder. Br J Psychiatry 2007;190:402–409.

6 Faraone SV, Perlis RH, Doyle AE, Smoller JW, Goralnick JJ, Holmgren MA, Sklar P: Molecular genetics if attention-deficit hyperactivity disorder. Biol Psychiatry 2005;57:1313–1323.

7 Comings DE, Chen TJ, Blum K, Mengucci JF, Blum SH, Meshkin B: Neurogenetic interactions and aberrant behavioral co-morbidity of attention-deficit hyperactivity disorder: dispelling myths. Theor Biol Med Model 2005;2:50–65.

8 American Psychiatric Association (APA): Diagnostic and Statistical Manual of Mental Disorders (Text Revision), ed 4. Washington, APA, 2000.

9 World Health Organization: International Statistical Classification of Diseases and Health-Related Problems. ICD-10, ed 2. Geneva, WHO, 1990.

10 Biederman J, Faraone SV, Keenan K, Benjamin J, Krifcher B, Moore C, Sprich-Buckminster S, Ugaglia K, Jellinek MS, Steingard R, et al: Further evidence for family-genetic risk factors in attention-deficit hyperactivity disorder. Patterns of comorbidity in probands and relatives psychiatrically and pediatrically referred samples. Arch Gen Psychiatry 1992;49: 728–738.

11 Faraone SV, Biederman J, Chen WJ, Milberger S, Warburton R, Tsuang MT: Genetic heterogeneity in attention-deficit hyperactivity disorder (ADHD): gender, psychiatric comorbidity, and maternal ADHD. J Abnorm Psychol 1995;104:334–345.

12 Faraone SV, Biederman J, Mennin D, Russell R, Tsuang MT: Familial subtypes of attention-deficit hyperactivity disorder: a 4-year follow-up study of children from antisocial ADHD families. J Child Psychol Psychiatry 1998;39:1045–1053.

13 Fisher SE, Francks C, McCracken JT, McGough JJ, Marlow AJ, MachPhie IL, Newbury DF, Crawford LR, Palmer CGS, Woodward JA, Del'Homme M, Cantwell DP, Nelson SF, Monaco AP, Smalley SL: A genomewide scan for loci involved in attention-deficit hyperactivity disorder. Am J Hum Genet 2002;70:1183–1196.

14 Smalley SL, Kustanovich V, Minassian SL, Stone JL, Ogdie MN, McGough JJ, McCracken JT, MacPhie IL, Francks C, Fisher SE, Cantor RM, Monaco AP, Nelson SF: Genetic linkage of attention-deficit hyperactivity disorder on chromosome 16p13, in a region implicated in autism. Am J Hum Genet 2002;71:959–963.

15 Arcos-Burgos M, Castellanos FX, Pineda D, Lopera F, Palacio JD, Palacio LG, Rapoport JL, Berg K, Bailey-Wilson JE, Muenke M: Attention-deficit hyperactivity disorder in a population isolate: linkage to loci at 4q13.2, 5q33.3, 11q22, and 17p11. Am J Hum Genet 2004;75:998–1014.

16 Bakker SC, van der Meulen EM, Buitelaar JK, Sandkuijl LA, Pauls DL, Monsuur AJ, van t'Slot R, Minderaa RB, Gunning WB, Pearson PL, Sinke RJ: A whole-genome scan in 164 Dutch sib pairs with attention-deficit hyperactivity disorder: suggestive evidence for linkage on chromosomes 7p and 15q. Am J Hum Genet 2003;72:1251–1260.

17 Ogdie MN, MacPhie IL, Minassian SL, Yang M, Fisher SE, Francks C, Cantor RM, McCracken JT, McGough JJ, Nelson SF, Monaco AP, Smalley SL: A genomewide scan for attention-deficit hyperactivity disorder in an extended sample: suggestive linkage on 17p11. Am J Hum Genet 2003;72:1268–1279.

18 Ogdie MN, Fisher SE, Yang M, Ishii J, Francks C, Loo SK, Cantor RM, McCracken JT, McGough JJ, Smalley SL, Nelson SF: Attention-deficit hyperactivity disorder: fine mapping supports linkage to 5p13, 6q12, 16p13, and 17p11. Am J Hum Genet 2004;75:661–668.

19 Hebebrand J, Dempfle A, Saar K, Thiele H, Herpertz-Dahlmann B, Linder M, Kiefl H, Remschmidt H, Hemminger U, Warnke A, Knölker U, Heiser P, Friedel S, Henney A, Schäfer H, Nürnberg P, Konrad K: A genome-wide scan for attention-deficit hyperactivity disorder in 155 German sib-pairs. Mol Psychiatry 2006;11:196–205.

20 Faraone SV, Doyle AE, Lasky-Su J, Sklar PB, D'Angelo E, Gonzalez-Heydrich J, Kratochvil C, Mick E, Klein K, Rezac AJ, Biederman J: Linkage analysis of attention-deficit hyperactivity disorder. Am J Med Genet B Neuropsychiatr Genet 2008; 147B:1387–1391.

21 Asherson P, Zhou K, Anney RJ, Franke B, Buitelaar J, Ebstein R, Gill M, Altink M, Arnold R, Boer F, Brookes K, Buschgens C, Butler L, Cambell D, Chen W, Christiansen H, Feldman L, Fleischman K, Fliers E, Howe-Forbes R, Goldfarb A, Heise A, Gabriëls I, Johansson L, Lubetzki I, Marco R, Medad S, Minderaa R, Mulas F, Müller U, Mulligan A, Neale B, Rijsdijk F, Rabin K, Rommelse N, Sethna V, Sorohan J, Uebel H, Psychogiou L, Weeks A, Barrett R, Xu X, Banaschewski T, Sonuga-Barke E, Eisenberg J, Manor I, Miranda A, Oades RD, Roeyers H, Rothenberger A, Sergeant J, Steinhausen HC, Taylor E, Thompson M, Faraone SV: A high-density SNP linkage scan with 142 combined subtype ADHD sib pairs identifies linkage regions on chromosomes 9 and 16. Mol Psychiatry 2008;13:514–521.

22 Romanos M, Freitag C, Jacob C, Craig DW, Dempfle A, Nguyen TT, Halperin R, Walitza S, Renner TJ, Seitz C, Romanos J, Palmason H, Reif A, Heine M, Windemuth-Kieselbach C, Vogler C, Sigmund J, Warnke A, Schäfer H, Meyer J, Stephan DA, Lesch KP: Genome-wide linkage analysis of ADHD using high-density SNP arrays: novel loci at 5q13.1 and 14q12. Mol Psychiatry 2008;13:522–530.

23 Amin N, Aulchenko YS, Dekker MC, Ferdinand RF, van Spreeken A, Temmink AH, Verhulst FC, Oostra BA, van Duijn CM: Suggestive linkage of ADHD to chromosome 18q22 in a young genetically isolated Dutch population. Eur J Hum Genet 2009; in press.

24 Friedel S, Saar K, Sauer S, Dempfle A, Walitza S, Renner T, Romanos M, Freitag C, Seitz C, Palmason H, Scherag A, Windemuth-Kieselbach C, Schimmelmann BG, Wewetzer C, Meyer J, Warnke A, Lesch KP, Reinhardt R, Herpertz-Dahlmann B, Linder M, Hinney A, Remschmidt H, Schäfer H, Konrad K, Hübner N, Hebebrand J: Association and linkage of allelic variants of the dopamine transporter gene in ADHD. Mol Psychiatry 2007;12:923–933.

25 Zhou K, Dempfle A, Arcos-Burgos M, Bakker SC, Banaschewski T, Biederman J, Buitelaar J, Castellanos FX, Doyle A, Ebstein RP, Ekholm J, Forabosco P, Franke B, Freitag C, Friedel S, Gill M, Hebebrand J, Hinney A, Jacob C, Lesch KP, Loo SK, Lopera F, McCracken JT, McGough JJ, Meyer J, Mick E, Miranda A, Muenke M, Mulas F, Nelson SF, Nguyen TT, Oades RD, Ogdie MN, Palacio JD, Pineda D, Reif A, Renner TJ, Roeyers H, Romanos M, Rothenberger A, Schäfer H, Sergeant J, Sinke RJ, Smalley SL, Sonuga-Barke E, Steinhausen HC, van der Meulen E, Walitza S, Warnke A, Lewis CM, Faraone SV, Asherson P: Meta-analysis of genome-wide linkage scans of attention-deficit hyperactivity disorder. Am J Med Genet B Neuropsychiatr Genet 2008;147B: 1392–1398.

26 Bobb AJ, Castellanos FX, Addington AM, Rapoport JL: Molecular genetic studies of ADHD: 1991–2004. Am J Med Genet B Neuropsychiatr Genet 2005; 132:109–125.

27 Albayrak O, Friedel S, Schimmelmann BG, Hinney A, Hebebrand J: Genetic aspects in attention-deficit hyperactivity disorder. J Neural Transm 2008;115: 305–315.

28 Waldman ID, Gizer IR: The genetics of attention-deficit hyperactivity disorder. Clin Psychol Rev 2006;26:396–432.

29 Gainetdinov RR, Wetsel WC, Jones SR, Levin ED, Jaber M, Caron MG: Role of serotonin in the paradoxical calming effect of psychostimulants on hyperactivity. Science 1999;283:397–402.

30 Heinz A, Goldman D, Jones DW, Palmour R, Hommer D, Gorey JG Lee KS, Linnoila M, Weinberger DR: Genotype influences in vivo dopamine transporter availability in human striatum. Neuropsychopharmacology 2000;22:133–139.

31 Jacobsen LK, Staley JK, Zoghbi SS, Seibyl JP, Kosten TR, Innis RB, Gelernter J: Prediction of dopamine transporter binding availability by genotype: a preliminary report. Am J Psychiatry 2000;157:1700–1703.

32 Dougherty DD, Bonab AA, Spencer TJ, Rauch SL, Madras BK, Fischman AJ: Dopamine transporter density is elevated in patients with ADHD. Lancet 1999;354:2132–2133.

33 Krause KH, Dresel SH, Krause J, Kung HF, Tatsch K: Increased striatal dopamine transporter in adult patients with attention-deficit hyperactivity disorder: effects of methylphenidate as measured by single photon emission computed tomography. Neurosci Lett 2000;285:107–110.

34 Cook EH Jr, Stein MA, Krasowski MD, Cox NJ, Olkon DM, Kieffer JE, Leventhal BL: Association of attention-deficit disorder and the dopamine transporter gene. Am J Hum Genet 1995;56:993–998.

35 Barr CL, Xu C, Kroft J, Feng Y, Wigg K, Zai G, Tannock R, Schachar R, Malone M, Roberts W, Nöthen MM, Grunhage F, Vandenbergh DJ, Uhl G, Sunohara G, King N, Kennedy JL: Haplotype study of three polymorphisms at the dopamine transporter locus confirm linkage to attention-deficit hyperactivity disorder. Biol Psychiatry 2001;49:333–339.

36 Hawi Z, Lowe N, Kirley A, Gruenhage F, Nothen M, Greenwood T, Kelsoe J, Fitzgerald M, Gill M: Linkage disequilibrium mapping at DAT1, DRD5 and DBH narrows the search for ADHD susceptibility alleles at these loci. Mol Psychiatry 2003;8:299–308.

37 Palmer CG, Bailey JN, Ramsey C, Cantwell D, Sinsheimer JS, Del'Homme M, McGough J, Woodward JA, Asarnow R, Asarnow J, Nelson S, Smalley SL: No evidence of linkage or linkage disequilibrium between DAT1 and attention-deficit hyperactivity disorder in a large sample. Psychiatr Genet 1999;9:157–160.

38 Holmes J, Payton A, Barrett JH, Hever T, Fitzpatrick H, Trumper AL, Harrington R, McGuffin P, Owen M, Ollier W, Worthington J, Thapar A: A family-based and case-control association study of the dopamine D4 receptor gene and dopamine transporter gene in attention-deficit hyperactivity disorder. Mol Psychiatry 2000;5:523–530.

39 Roman T, Schmitz M, Polanczyk GV, Eizirik M, Rohde LA, Hutz MH: Attention-deficit hyperactivity disorder: a study of association with both the dopamine transporter gene and the dopamine D4 receptor gene. Am J Med Genet 2001;105:471–478.

40 Li D, Sham PC, Owen MJ, He L: Meta-analysis shows significant association between dopamine system genes and attention-deficit hyperactivity disorder. Hum Mol Genet 2006;15:2276–2284.

41 Maher BS, Marazita ML, Ferrell RE, Vanyukov MM: Dopamine system genes and attention-deficit hyperactivity disorder: a meta-analysis. Psychiatr Genet 2002;12:207–215.

42 Curran S, Mill J, Tahir E, Kent L, Richards S, Gould A, Huckett L, Sharp J, Batten C, Fernando S, Ozbay F, Yazgan Y, Simonoff E, Thompson M, Taylor E, Asherson P: Association study of a dopamine transporter polymorphism and attention-deficit hyperactivity disorder in UK and Turkish samples. Mol Psychiatry 2001;6:425–428.

43 Kirley A, Lowe N, Hawi Z, Mullins C, Daly G, Waldman I, McCarron M, O'Donnell D, Fitzgerald M, Gill M: Association of the 480 bp DAT1 allele with methylphenidate response in a sample of Irish children with ADHD. Am J Med Genet B Neuropsychiatr Genet 2003;121:50–54.

44 Joober R, Grizenko N, Sengupta S, Amor LB, Schmitz N, Schwartz G, Karama S, Lageix P, Fathalli F, Torkaman-Zehi A, Stepanian MT: Dopamine transporter 3′-UTR VNTR genotype and ADHD: pharmaco-behavioural genetic study with methylphenidate. Neuropsychopharmacology 2007;32:1370–1376.

45 Stein MA, Waldman ID, Sarampote CS, Seymour KE, Robb AS, Conlon C, Kim SJ, Cook EH: Dopamine transporter genotype and methylphenidate dose response in children with ADHD. Neuropsychopharmacology 2005;30:1374–1382.

46 Van der Meulen EM, Bakker SC, Pauls DL, Oteman N, Kruitwagen CL, Pearson PL, Sinke RJ, Buitelaar JK: High sibling correlation on methylphenidate response but no association with DAT1-10R homozygosity in Dutch sib pairs with ADHD. J Child Psychol Psychiatry 2005;46:1074–1080.

47 Mick E, Biederman J, Spencer T, Faraone SV, Sklar P: Absence of association with DST1 polymorphism and response to methylphenidate in a sample of adults with ADHD. Am J Med Genet B Neuropsychiatr Genet 2006;141:890–894.

48 Barkley RA, Smith KM, Fischer M, Navia B: An examination of the behavioral and neuropsychological correlates of three ADHD candidate gene polymorphisms (DRD4 7+, DBH TaqI A2, and DAT1 40 bp VNTR) in hyperactive and normal children followed to adulthood. Am J Med Genet B Neuropsychiatr Genet 2006;141:487–498.

49 Ebstein RP, Novick O, Umansky R, Priel B, Osher Y, Blaine D, Bennett ER, Nemanov L, Katz M, Belmaker RH: Dopamine D4 receptor (D4DR) exon III polymorphism associated with the human personality trait of novelty seeking. Nat Genet 1996;12:78–80.

50 Durston S, Fossella JA, Casey BJ, Hulshoff Pol HE, Galvan A, Schnack HG, Steenhuis MP, Minderaa RB, Buitelaar JK, Kahn RS, van Engeland H: Differential effects of DRD4 and DAT1 genotype on fronto-striatal gray matter volumes in a sample of subjects with attention-deficit hyperactivity disorder, their unaffected siblings, and controls. Mol Psychiatry 2005;10:678–685.

51 LaHoste GJ, Swanson JM, Wigal SB, Glabe C, Wigal T, King N, Kennedy JL: Dopamine D4 receptor gene polymorphism is associated with attention-deficit hyperactivity disorder. Mol Psychiatry 1996;1:121–124.

52 Holmes J, Payton A, Barrett J, Harrington R, McGuffin P, Owen M, Ollier W, Worthington J, Gill M, Kirley A, Hawi Z, Fitzgerald M, Asherson P, Curran S, Mill J, Gould A, Taylor E, Kent L, Craddock N, Thapar A: Association of DRD4 in children with ADHD and comorbid conduct problems. Am J Med Genet 2002;114:150–153.

53 Gornick MC, Addington A, Shaw P, Bobb AJ, Sharp W, Greenstein D, Arepalli S, Castellanos FX, Rapoport JL: Association of the dopamine receptor D4 (DRD4) gene 7-repeat allele with children with attention-deficit hyperactivity disorder: an update. Am J Med Genet B Neuropsychiatr Genet 2007;144B:379–382.

54 Birkas E, Lakatos K, Nemoda Z, Ney K, Toth I, Novak A, Sasvari-Szekely M, Gervai J: Effects of the D4 dopamine receptor gene variation on behavior problems at 6 years of age (in Hungarian). Neuropsychopharmacol Hung 2005;7:125–131.

55 Grady DL, Chi HC, Ding YC, Smith M, Wang E, Schuck S, Flodman P, Spence MA, Swanson JM, Moyzis RK: High prevalence of rare dopamine receptor D4 alleles in children diagnosed with attention-deficit hyperactivity disorder. Mol Psychiatry 2003;8:536–545.

56 Lowe N, Kirley A, Mullins C, Fitzgerald M, Gill M, Hawi Z: Multiple marker analysis at the promoter region of the DRD4 gene and ADHD: evidence of linkage and association with the SNP-616. Am J Med Genet B Neuropsychiatr Genet 2004;131:33–37.

57 Kereszturi E, Kiraly O, Csapo Z, Tarnok Z, Gadoros J, Sasvari-Szekely M, Nemoda Z: Association between the 120-bp duplication of the dopamine D4 receptor gene and attention-deficit hyperactivity disorder: genetic and molecular analyses. Am J Med Genet B Neuropsychiatr Genet 2007;144B:231–236.

58 Faraone SV, Doyle AE, Mick E, Biederman J: Meta-analysis of the association between the 7-repeat allele of the dopamine D4 receptor gene and attention-deficit hyperactivity disorder. Am J Psychiatry 2001;158:1052–1057.

59 Egger M, Davey Smith G, Schneider M, Minder C: Bias in meta-analysis detected by a simple, graphical test. BMJ 1997;315:629–634.

60 Daly G, Hawi Z, Fitzgerald M, Gill M: Mapping susceptibility loci in attention-deficit hyperactivity disorder: preferential transmission of parental alleles at DAT1, DBH and DRD5 to affected children. Mol Psychiatry 1999;4:192–196.

61 Lowe N, Kirley A, Hawi Z, Sham P, Wickham H, Kratochvil CJ, Smith SD, Lee SY, Levy F, Kent L, Middle F, Rohde LA, Roman T, Tahir E, Yazgan Y, Asherson P, Mill J, Thapar A, Payton A, Todd RD, Stephens T, Ebstein RP, Manor I, Barr CL, Wigg KG, Sinke RJ, Buitelaar JK, Smalley SL, Nelson SF, Biederman J, Faraone SV, Gill M: Joint analysis of the DRD5 marker concludes association with attention-deficit hyperactivity disorder confined to the predominantly inattentive and combined subtypes. Am J Hum Genet 2004;74:348–356.

62 Tang Y, Buxbaum SG, Waldman I, Anderson GM, Zabetian CP, Kohnke MD, Cubells JF: A single nucleotide polymorphism at DBH, possibly associated with attention-deficit hyperactivity disorder, associates with lower plasma dopamine β-hydroxylase activity and is in linkage disequilibrium with two putative functional single nucleotide polymorphisms. Biol Psychiatry 2006;60:1034–1038.

63 Roman T, Schmitz M, Polanczyk GV, Eizirik M, Rohde LA, Hutz MH: Further evidence for the association between attention-deficit hyperactivity disorder and the dopamine β-hydroxylase gene. Am J Med Genet 2002;114:154–158.

64 Wigg K, Zai G, Schachar R, Tannock R, Roberts W, Malone M, Kennedy JL, Barr CL: Attention-deficit hyperactivity disorder and the gene for dopamine β-hydroxylase. Am J Psychiatry 2002;159:1046–1048.

65 Inkster B, Muglia P, Jain U, Kennedy JL: Linkage disequilibrium analysis of the dopamine β-hydroxylase gene in persistent attention-deficit hyperactivity disorder. Psychiatr Genet 2004;14:117–120.

66 Bhaduri N, Sinha S, Chattopadhyay A, Gangopadhyay PK, Singh M, Mukhopadhyay KK: Analysis of polymorphisms in the dopamine β-hydroxylase gene: association with attention deficit hyperactivity disorder in Indian children. Indian Pediatr 2005;42: 123–129.

67 Barr CL, Kroft J, Feng Y, Wigg K, Roberts W, Malone M, Ickowicz A, Schachar R, Tannock R, Kennedy JL: The norepinephrine transporter gene and attention-deficit hyperactivity disorder. Am J Med Genet 2002;114:255–259.

68 McEvoy B, Hawi Z, Fitzgerald M, Gill M: No evidence of linkage or association between the norepinephrine transporter gene polymorphisms and ADHD in the Irish population. Am J Med Genet 2002;114:665–666.

69 De Luca V, Muglia P, Jain U, Kennedy JL: No evidence of linkage or association between the norepinephrine transporter gene MnlI polymorphism and adult ADHD. Am J Med Genet B Neuropsychiatr Genet 2004;124:38–40.

70 Bobb AJ, Addington AM, Sidransky E, Gornick MC, Lerch JP, Greenstein DK, Clasen LS, Sharp WS, Inoff-Germain G, Wavrant-De Vrieze F, Arcos-Burgos M, Straub RE, Hardy JA, Castellanos FX, Rapoport JL: Support for association between ADHD and two candidate genes: NET1 and DRD1. Am J Med Genet B Neuropsychiatr Genet 2005;134: 67–72.

71 Xu X, Knight J, Brookes K, Mill J, Sham P, Craig I, Taylor E, Asherson P: DNA pooling analysis of 21 norepinephrine transporter gene SNPs with attention-deficit hyperactivity disorder: no evidence for association. Am J Med Genet B Neuropsychiatr Genet 2005;134:115–118.

72 Kim CH, Hahn MK, Joung Y, Anderson SL, Steele AH, Mazei-Robinson MS, Gizer I, Teicher MH, Cohen BM, Robertson D, Waldman ID, Blakely RD, Kim KS: A polymorphism in the norepinephrine transporter gene alters promoter activity and is associated with attention-deficit hyperactivity disorder. Proc Natl Acad Sci USA 2006;103:19164–19169.

73 Yang L, Wang YF, Li J, Faraone SV: Association of norepinephrine transporter gene with methylphenidate response. J Am Acad Child Adolesc Psychiatry 2004;43:1154–1158.

74 Comings DE, Gade-Andavolu R, Gonzalez N, Blake H, Wu S, MacMurray JP: Additive effect of three noradrenergic genes (ADRA2a, ADRA2c, DBH) on attention-deficit hyperactivity disorder and learning disabilities in Tourette syndrome subjects. Clin Genet 1999;55:160–172.

75 Barr CL, Wigg K, Zai G, Roberts W, Malone M, Schachar R, Tannock R, Kennedy JL: Attention-deficit hyperactivity disorder and the adrenergic receptors α1C and α2C. Mol Psychiatry 2001;6:334–337.

76 Xu C, Schachar R, Tannock R, Roberts W, Malone M, Kennedy JL, Barr CL: Linkage study of the α2A adrenergic receptor in attention-deficit hyperactivity disorder families. Am J Med Genet 2001;105:159–162.

77 Levitan RD, Masellis M, Basile VS, Lam RW, Jain U, Kaplan AS, Kennedy SH, Siegel G, Walker ML, Vaccarino FJ, Kennedy JL: Polymorphism of the serotonin-2A receptor gene (HTR2A) associated with childhood attention-deficit hyperactivity disorder in adult women with seasonal affective disorder. J Affect Disord 2002;71:229–233.
78 Roman T, Schmitz M, Polanczyk GV, Eizirik M, Rohde LA, Hutz MH: Is the α2A adrenergic receptor gene (ADRA2A) associated with attention-deficit hyperactivity disorder? Am J Med Genet B Neuropsychiatr Genet 2003;120:116–120.
79 Retz W, Retz-Junginger P, Supprian T, Thome J, Rösler M: Association of serotonin promoter gene polymorphism with violence: relation with personality disorders, impulsivity and childhood ADHD psychopathology. Behav Sci Law 2004;22:415–425.
80 Seeger G, Schloss P, Schmidt MH: Functional polymorphism within the promoter of the serotonin transporter gene is associated with severe hyperkinetic disorders. Mol Psychiatry 2001;6:235–238.
81 Retz W, Thome J, Blocher D, Baader M, Rösler M: Association of attention-deficit hyperactivity disorder-related psychopathology and personality traits with the serotonin transporter promoter region polymorphism. Neurosci Lett 2002;319:133–136.
82 Manor I, Eisenberg J, Tyano S, Sever Y, Cohen H, Ebstein RP, Kotler M: Family-based association study of the serotonin transporter promoter region polymorphism (5-HTTLPR) in attention-deficit hyperactivity disorder. Am J Med Genet 2001;105: 91–95.
83 Zoroglu SS, Erdal ME, Alasehirli B, Erdal N, Sivasli E, Tutkun H, Savas HA, Herken H: Significance of serotonin transporter gene 5-HTTLPR and variable number of tandem repeat polymorphism in attention-deficit hyperactivity disorder. Neuropsychobiology 2002;47:17–20.
84 Beitchman JH, Davidge KM, Kennedy JL, Atkinson L, Lee V, Shapiro S, Douglas L: The serotonin transporter gene in aggressive children with and without ADHD and nonaggressive matched controls. Ann NY Acad Sci 2003;1008:248–251.
85 Kent L, Doerry U, Hardy E, Parmar R, Gingell K, Hawi Z, Kirley A, Lowe N, Fitzgerald M, Gill M, Craddock N: Evidence that variation at the serotonin transporter gene influences susceptibility to attention-deficit hyperactivity disorder (ADHD): analysis and pooled analysis. Mol Psychiatry 2002;7: 908–912.
86 Curran S, Purcell S, Craig I, Asherson P, Sham P: The serotonin transporter gene as a QTL for ADHD. Am J Med Genet B Neuropsychiatr Genet 2005;134: 42–47.
87 Li J, Wang Y, Zhou R, Zhang H, Yang L, Wang B, Faraone SV: Association between polymorphisms in serotonin transporter gene and attention-deficit hyperactivity disorder in Chinese Han subjects. Am J Med Genet B Neuropsychiatr Genet 2007;144:14–19.
88 Cadoret RJ, Langbehn D, Caspers K, Troughton EP, Yucuis R, Sandhu HK, Philibert R: Associations of the serotonin transporter promoter polymorphism with aggressivity, attention deficit, and conduct disorder in an adoptee population. Compr Psychiatry 2003;44:88–101.
89 Kim SJ, Badner J, Cheon KA, Kim BN, Yoo HJ, Kim SJ, Cook E Jr, Leventhal BL, Kim YS: Family-based association study of the serotonin transporter gene polymorphisms in Korean ADHD trios. Am J Med Genet B Neuropsychiatr Genet 2005;139:14–18.
90 Xu X, Mill J, Chen CK, Brookes K, Taylor E, Asherson P: Family-based association study of serotonin transporter gene polymorphism in attention-deficit hyperactivity disorder: no evidence for association in UK and Taiwanese samples. Am J Med Genet B Neuropsychiatr Genet 2005;139:11–13.
91 Langley K, Payton A, Hamshere ML, Pay HM, Lawson DC, Turic D, Ollier W, Worthington J, Owen MJ, O'Donovan MC, Thapar A: No evidence of association of two 5-HT transporter gene polymorphisms and attention-deficit hyperactivity disorder. Psychiatr Genet 2003;13:107–110.
92 Zhao AL, Su LY, Zhang YH, Tang BS, Luo XR, Huang CX, Su QR: Association analysis of serotonin transporter promoter gene polymorphism with ADHD and related symptomatology. Int J Neurosci 2005;115:1183–1191.
93 Heiser P, Dempfle A, Friedel S, Konrad K, Hinney A, Kiefl H, Walitza S, Bettecken T, Saar K, Linder M, Warnke A, Herpertz-Dahlmann B, Schäfer H, Remschmidt H, Hebebrand J: Family-based association study of serotonergic candidate genes and attention-deficit hyperactivity disorder in a German sample. J Neural Transm 2007;114:513–521.
94 Wigg KG, Takhar A, Ickowicz A, Tannock R, Kennedy JL, Pathare T, Malone M, Schachar R, Barr CL: Gene for the serotonin transporter and ADHD: no association with two functional polymorphisms. Am J Med Genet B Neuropsychiatr Genet 2006;141: 566–570.
95 Zoroglu SS, Erdal ME, Erdal N, Ozen S, Alasehirli B, Sivasli E: No evidence for an association between the T102C and 1438 G/A polymorphisms of the serotonin 2A receptor gene in attention-deficit hyperactivity disorder in a Turkish population. Neuropsychobiology 2003;47:17–20.

96 Quist JF, Barr CL, Schachar R, Roberts W, Malone M, Tannock R, Basile VS, Beitchman J, Kennedy JL: Evidence for the serotonin HTR2A receptor gene as a susceptibility factor in attention-deficit hyperactivity disorder. Mol Psychiatry 2000;5:537–541.
97 Hawi Z, Dring M, Kirley A, Foley D, Kent L, Craddock N, Asherson P, Curran S, Gould A, Richards S, Lawson D, Pay H, Turic D, Langley K, Owen M, O'Donovan M, Thapar A, Fitzgerald M, Gill M: Serotonergic system and attention-deficit hyperactivity disorder: a potential susceptibility locus at the 5-HT_{1B} receptor gene in 273 nuclear families from a multicentre sample. Mol Psychiatry 2002;7:718–725.
98 Walitza S, Renner TJ, Dempfle A, Konrad K, Wewetzer C, Halbach A, Herpertz-Dahlmann B, Remschmidt H, Smidt J, Linder M, Flierl L, Knolker U, Friedel S, Schäfer H, Gross C, Hebebrand J, Warnke A, Lesch KP: Transmission disequilibrium of polymorphic variants in the tryptophan hydroxylase-2 gene in attention-deficit hyperactivity disorder. Mol Psychiatry 2005;10:1126–1132.
99 Sheehan K, Lowe N, Kirley A, Mullins C, Fitzgerald M, Gill M, Hawi Z: Tryptophan hydroxylase-2 gene variants associated with ADHD. Mol Psychiatry 2005;10:944–949.
100 Brookes K, Xu X, Chen W, Zhou K, Neale B, Lowe N, Anney R, Franke B, Gill M, Ebstein R, Buitelaar J, Sham P, Campbell D, Knight J, Andreou P, Altink M, Arnold R, Boer F, Buschgens C, Butler L, Christiansen H, Feldman L, Fleischman K, Fliers E, Howe-Forbes R, Goldfarb A, Heise A, Gabriels I, Korn-Lubetzki I, Johansson L, Marco R, Medad S, Minderaa R, Mulas F, Muller U, Mulligan A, Rabin K, Rommelse N, Sethna V, Sorohan J, Uebel H, Psychogiou L, Weeks A, Barrett R, Craig I, Banaschewski T, Sonuga-Barke E, Eisenberg J, Kuntsi J, Manor I, McGuffin P, Miranda A, Oades RD, Plomin R, Roeyers H, Rothenberger A, Sergeant J, Steinhausen HC, Taylor E, Thompson M, Faraone SV, Asherson P: The analysis of 51 genes in DSM-IV combined type attention-deficit hyperactivity disorder: association signals in DRD4, DAT1 and 16 other genes. Mol Psychiatry 2006;11:934–953.
101 Sheehan K, Hawi Z, Gill M, Kent L: No association between TPH2 gene polymorphisms and ADHD in a UK sample. Neurosci Lett 2007;412:105–107.
102 Neale BM, Lasky-Su J, Anney R, Franke B, Zhou K, Maller JB, Vasquez AA, Asherson P, Chen W, Banaschewski T, Buitelaar J, Ebstein R, Gill M, Miranda A, Oades RD, Roeyers H, Rothenberger A, Sergeant J, Steinhausen HC, Sonuga-Barke E, Mulas F, Taylor E, Laird N, Lange C, Daly M, Faraone SV: Genome-wide association scan of attention-deficit hyperactivity disorder. Am J Med Genet B Neuropsychiatr Genet 2008;147B:1337–1344.
103 Lasky-Su J, Anney RJ, Neale BM, Franke B, Zhou K, Maller JB, Vasquez AA, Chen W, Asherson P, Buitelaar J, Banaschewski T, Ebstein R, Gill M, Miranda A, Mulas F, Oades RD, Roeyers H, Rothenberger A, Sergeant J, Sonuga-Barke E, Steinhausen HC, Taylor E, Daly M, Laird N, Lange C, Faraone SV: Genome-wide association scan of the time to onset of attention-deficit hyperactivity disorder. Am J Med Genet B Neuropsychiatr Genet 2008;147B:1355–1358.
104 Lesch KP, Timmesfeld N, Renner TJ, Halperin R, Röser C, Nguyen TT, Craig DW, Romanos J, Heine M, Meyer J, Freitag C, Warnke A, Romanos M, Schäfer H, Walitza S, Reif A, Stephan DA, Jacob C: Molecular genetics of adult ADHD: converging evidence from genome-wide association and extended pedigree linkage studies. J Neural Transm 2008;115:1573–1585.
105 Thapar A, Harrington R, McGuffin P: Examining the comorbidity of ADHD-related behaviours and conduct problems using a twin study design. Br J Psychiatry 2001;179:224–229.
106 Langley K, Rice F, van den Bree MB, Thapar A: Maternal smoking during pregnancy as an environmental risk factor for attention-deficit hyperactivity disorder behaviour. A review. Minerva Pediatr 2005;57:359–371.
107 Bhutta AT, Cleves MA, Casey PH, Cradock MM, Anand KJ: Cognitive and behavioral outcomes of school-aged children who were born preterm: a meta-analysis. JAMA 2002;288:728–737.
108 Blanz B, Schmidt MH, Esser G: Familial adversities and child psychiatric disorders. J Child Psychol Psychiat 1991;32:939–950.
109 Fergusson DM, Lynskey MT, Horwood LJ: Factors associated with continuity and changes in disruptive behaviour patterns between childhood and adolescence. J Abnorm Child Psychol 1996;24:533–553.
110 Rutter M: Psychosocial adversity and child psychopathology. Br J Psychiatry 1999;174:480–493.
111 Biederman J, Milberger S, Faraone SV, Kiely K, Guite J, Mick E, Ablon S, Warburton R, Reed E: Family-environment risk factors for attention-deficit hyperactivity disorder. A test of Rutter's indicators of adversity. Arch Gen Psychiatry 1995;52:464–470.
112 Khan RS, Khoury J, Nichols WC, Lanphear BP: Role of dopamine transporter genotype and maternal prenatal smoking in childhood hyperactive-impulsive, inattentive and oppositional behaviours. J Pediatr 2003;143:104–110.
113 Becker K, El-Faddagh M, Schmidt MH, Esser G, Laucht M: Interaction of dopamine transporter genotype with prenatal smoke exposure on ADHD symptoms. J Pediatr. 2008;152:263–269.

114 Retz W, Freitag CM, Retz-Junginger P, Wenzler D, Schneider M, Kissling C, Thome J, Rösler M: A functional serotonin transporter promoter gene polymorphism increases ADHD symptoms in delinquents: interaction with adverse childhood environment. Psychiatry Res 2008;158:123–131.

115 Müller DJ, Mandelli L, Serretti A, DeYoung CG, De Luca V, Sicard T, Tharmalingam S, Gallinat J, Muglia P, De Ronchi D, Jain U, Kennedy JL: Serotonin transporter gene and adverse life events in adult ADHD. Am J Med Genet B Neuropsychiatr Genet 2008;147B:1461–1469.

Prof. Wolfgang Retz, MD
Saarland University Hospital, Institute for Forensic Psychology and Psychiatry
DE–66421 Homburg/Saar (Germany)
Tel. +49 6841 1626350, Fax +49 6841 1626335, E-Mail wolfgang.retz@uniklinik-saarland.de

Retz W, Klein RG (eds): Attention-Deficit Hyperactivity Disorder (ADHD) in Adults.
Key Issues in Mental Health. Basel, Karger, 2010, vol 176, pp 78–87

Neurophysiology of Adult Attention-Deficit Hyperactivity Disorder

Christina G. Baehne · Andreas J. Fallgatter

Department of Psychiatry and Psychotherapy, University of Würzburg, Würzburg, Germany

Abstract

Electrophysiological studies in adult attention-deficit hyperactivity disorder (ADHD) patients are still very sparse. Therefore, the first part of the chapter shortly reviews quantitative EEG (qEEG) as well as event-related potential (ERP) studies in children with ADHD. Basically, ADHD children are characterized by a slowing in their qEEG frequencies and by longer latencies and smaller amplitudes in some (but not all) of the ERP components. Generally, neurophysiological impairments described in the few studies on adult ADHD patients are very similar to those of children with ADHD, while others change with age and, therefore, might present a developmental perspective. A promising approach for future studies may be the search for distinct subtypes or endophenotypes in ADHD which can be detected with the help of EEG parameters. This strategy may be useful for the development of more individualized and efficient treatments.

Electrophysiology

This chapter provides an overview of electrophysiological investigations in attention-deficit hyperactivity disorder (ADHD) patients. While ADHD-like symptomatology in children was already diagnosed in the early 1900s (under different diagnostic concepts), this disease was not recognized in adults until the 1970s [1]. DSM-IV was the first classification manual that also accepted the diagnosis of ADHD in adulthood. While DSM-IV describes predominantly inattentive, predominantly hyperactive and combined subtypes of ADHD, the ICD-10 classification regards the presence of hyperactivity as essential for the diagnosis. This is not adequate for the situation in adult ADHD patients, who frequently do not show a clear-cut hyperactive symptomatology [1]. The relatively short time span that adult ADHD has been in the focus of psychiatric research may explain why there is a burgeoning literature in

Supported by the Deutsche Forschungsgemeinschaft (KFO 125/1-1).

electrophysiological investigations in ADHD children but only a few investigations in adult ADHD patients. Nonetheless, until today, ADHD diagnosis in children as in adults is hampered by the fact that objective diagnostic measures are missing. Like for most other psychiatric disorders, the diagnosis of ADHD has to rely above all on subjective judgments of parents, teachers, self-reports, and the clinical assessment. Adults have to retrospectively recall their childhood symptomatology as it is a necessity for the diagnosis that the disorder was already present in childhood before the age of 7 years. Moreover, the diagnostic criteria listed in the classification manuals are mainly created for children, and are not adapted to the adult situation.

ADHD research in the past has furthermost focused on behavioral and performance abnormalities, which show a large overlap with the healthy population. Therefore, the interest in the neural basis of the clinically relevant behavioral abnormalities grew steadily and is still a major focus in ADHD research. The search for brain activation patterns that may be an indicator for this disorder is heavily going on, applying different electrophysiological and brain-imaging techniques. Neurophysiological measures may bring additional insights into the pathophysiology underlying ADHD, and may be considered as endophenotypes closer correlated with the fundamental genetic abnormalities than the behavior and the clinical symptoms themselves.

One method to measure neural mechanisms in ADHD is electroencephalography (EEG). EEG is a method that measures brain potential fluctuations at the surface of the scalp. At least two electrodes are required to measure the electrical potentials. These potentials are created by simultaneously active neuronal cell assemblies in the brain. EEG is a relatively cheap method (compared to other imaging techniques like PET, SPECT or MRI), has no risk and is not invasive. It has been proven to be a suitable tool to detect differences between ADHD patients and controls. The search for specific neural abnormalities in ADHD has generated a large body of EEG research in children with ADHD either in the domain of quantitative EEG (qEEG) or event-related potentials (ERPs). In children with ADHD, most often an increase in low-frequency activity (i.e. theta) and a decrease in high-frequency activity (i.e. beta and alpha) compared with age-matched controls was detected [2]. This is in line with the view that an impairment of the regulation of activation in the central nervous system is fundamental in ADHD. In ERP studies (during oddball tasks, continuous performance tests) higher N100 amplitudes and lower P300 amplitudes as well as sometimes longer P300 latencies in children with ADHD were found, but results are task-dependent [3, 4]. Therefore, a higher initial orienting reaction (higher N100 amplitudes), energetic deficits in the processing of a target (lower posterior P300 amplitudes), and a delay in processing (longer latencies) can be assumed in ADHD children. Moreover, a normalization of disturbed EEG patterns under medication was described [5–8]. As EEG activity systematically changes with age, it is not appropriate to infer the same abnormalities in adults like in children. EEG profiles have to be investigated also in adults with ADHD and compared with the pattern in adult control participants.

Quantitative EEG (qEEG)

The EEG can be dissected in the different frequency bands (commonly alpha 8–13 Hz, beta 13.5–30 Hz, theta 4–7.5 Hz, delta 0.5–3.5 Hz). The absolute (total power) or the relative power (ratio) of the respective frequency band can be analyzed. The dominant EEG frequency band depends on the activity state of the person under investigation. The EEG of healthy adults in a resting state with eyes closed is usually characterized by alpha activity with a center of gravity over parietal and occipital brain areas. In the transition to sleep, theta and delta activity is increasing. However, EEG frequency in awake states also reflects developmental processes of the brain from newborns to adults with basic EEG frequencies increasing steadily from delta to alpha.

In ADHD children, the resting state EEG is characterized by more slow wave activity as compared to healthy children of the same age [2]. The most common findings are elevated theta power, and reduced alpha and/or beta power, as well as an increase in theta/alpha and/or theta/beta ratio. These observations could be indicators of reduced arousal in ADHD children as activation and arousal of the central nervous system is reflected in the firing patterns of neurons. Generally, higher frequencies reflect alert and aroused mental states, while lower frequencies suggest inattentiveness.

qEEG also is a useful tool to map responses to different conditions/stimuli or the performance in different tasks [9]. To date, qEEG studies with adult ADHD patients are scarce. Monastra et al. [9] measured 482 participants, consisting of ADHD patients of the inattentive and combined subtypes and healthy controls in the age range from 6 to 30 years. They used only a single electrode at the vertex with the earlobes as reference. The participants were measured in an eyes-open resting condition, while silently reading, listening, or drawing. For each task the calculation of the theta/beta power ratio was performed. qEEG findings indicated an age effect on basic EEG frequencies, with higher ratios in younger participants. The theta/beta power ratio was significantly elevated in ADHD patients compared to healthy controls irrespective of the clinical subtype in all tasks. In the ADHD groups, higher theta/beta power ratios were found in the drawing task as compared to the other tasks. The drawing task was the only task where significant differences in power ratios emerged between the combined and the inattentive ADHD subtypes. Bresnahan et al. [10] analyzed the frequency bands delta, theta, alpha, and beta at midline electrode sites (Fz, Cz, Pz) in an eyes-open resting condition in 25 children (6–11 years), 25 adolescents (13–17 years), and 25 adults (20–42 years) with ADHD of the combined subtype and without comorbid disorders and the same number of healthy controls for each group. ADHD patients showed elevated slow wave activity (absolute and relative theta and delta) in all age groups as compared to healthy controls. In contrast, no differences either in absolute and relative alpha or in absolute beta power were found between healthy controls and ADHD. Moreover, the theta/beta ratio was increased in ADHD. Generally, ADHD groups showed less fast wave but more slow wave activity. The ADHD patients had higher total power than the healthy controls with decreasing values for both groups with age. These results are well in line with previous findings in children. Furthermore, relative beta power was decreased in ADHD patients, but this reduction decreased systematically with age. At Fz and Cz a normalization with age emerged, but the relative beta power stayed decreased at Pz. As the hyperactive ADHD symptomatology also tends to decreases with age, the authors suggested that in ADHD patients the reduced beta activity in frontal and central sites might be related to behavioral hyperactivity symptoms. Moreover, the authors hypothesized that the increase of theta activity found in adults as well as in children with ADHD might reflect impulsive behavior, which frequently persists in adult ADHD. In order to further investigate the specificity of these findings in adults, Bresnahan and Barry [11] compared the EEG profiles during an eyes-open resting condition in 50 adult ADHD patients with those of 50 patients with some ADHD symptoms but no full diagnosis (subclinical ADHD) and 50 healthy controls. Taken together, absolute and relative theta was elevated in ADHD patients compared to the subclinical ADHD group and also to the healthy control group. Relative theta was reduced and relative beta power was increased in the subclinical ADHD group as compared to the ADHD and healthy control group. This differential finding may serve to separate the diagnostic groups and is in line with the former study [11].

In another study this research group reported that treatment with the stimulant dexamphetamine was followed by an amelioration of the clinical symptomatology and also by a normalization of the EEG profile consisting of a reduction of absolute delta, absolute and relative theta and total power in 50 ADHD patients who responded to the medication [12]. However, with respect to absolute and relative theta, the normalization was incomplete and the authors hypothesized that these still deviant EEG patterns may be related to residual symptoms still detectable in patients under medication.

In order to elucidate psychophysiological mechanisms in adult ADHD, Hermens et al. [13] investigated the skin conductance level (as an index of arousal) and qEEG during an eyes-closed resting condition. The study was designed to detect differences between adults with ADHD and healthy controls and also to investigate sex differences in ADHD patients. 21 male and 14 female adults with ADHD and age- and gender-matched controls were included. The authors found deviations in qEEG from normal controls (increased theta and delta activity and decreased beta (posterior region)) and skin conductance level (decreased skin conductance) in ADHD adults. A closer look at gender differences revealed different findings for men and women. The increased theta activity that was found in the whole ADHD group was due to the pronounced increase of theta in ADHD men. The decreased skin conductance however depended on a stronger decrease in ADHD females (hypoarousal). The authors interpreted their findings as a hint for different etiological mechanisms of ADHD in men and women.

A study of Philipsen et al. [14] in which qEEG during sleep was investigated could not find any differences in adult ADHD patients (combined subtype) without any personality disorder or actual major depressive disorder or substance abuse/dependency compared to healthy controls. The patients did not take any psychotropic medication for at least 2 weeks before assessment. Nonetheless, during sleep the motor activity was elevated and the subjective rating of sleep quality was decreased in the patient group as compared to healthy controls. These results give reason to speculate that differences in EEG frequencies between adult ADHD patients and healthy controls are only observable when participants are awake and therefore they should only be investigated in an alert state. In a state when both groups are expected to have low arousal (sleep), no differences emerged.

Event-Related Potentials

The ERPs recorded from the scalp may be considered as a synchronized part of the pattern of ongoing electroencephalogram. Endogenous as well as exogenous events elicit stimulus locked voltage fluctuations that can be measured with an ongoing EEG from the scalp. After filtering and averaging a number of at least 20 stimulus-locked EEG segments, the resulting ERPs depict the voltage changes elicited by a particular event class in the time domain. Averaging of the data is necessary to reduce the noise portion that adds to the signal and therefore to improve the signal-to-noise ratio. ERPs reflect aspects of the stimulus material as well as aspects of the stimulus processing within the individual brain. The excellent time resolution of EEG-based methods allows unrevealing the time course of different processes involved in the evaluation of a given stimulus. In contrast, the spatial resolution of EEG-based methods is rather poor. An ERP typically has a waveform consisting of positive and negative peaks. These peaks can be described with the amplitude (height, μV) of the waves as well as with the latency (timing, ms) of the peaks. The amplitude reflects the number of simultaneously active neurons (magnitude of activation) while the latency reflects the time course of the underlying process. More sophisticated analysis methods are for example topographical analyses of the positive or negative brain electrical fields, area measurements, multivariate analysis methods like principal component analysis, or source location analyses [15, 16].

Early ERP components are deflections within the first 100 ms after the stimulus. They are dependent on stimulus characteristics (modality, intensity, etc.) as well as on the integrity of neuronal transmission processes. They are therefore called *exogenous potentials*. Potentials from about 100 ms on are not only dependent on the physical properties of the stimulus and intact signal transmission processes but also on psychological processes. They are therefore denoted as *endogenous components*. Controlled and conscious processing of stimuli is reflected in components from 150–200 ms on. Changes in neural activity reflecting cognitive processing are related to task demands and often appear in a range of about 300 ms after presentation (P300) [15]. For the calculation of ERPs, only correct (or only false) answers should be averaged. This is helpful in determining whether different processing strategies or brain structures are involved in the same task in different groups of individuals. So ERPs offer a unique possibility to measure the effect of an experimental manipulation on brain activity patterns. With ERPs more subtle changes or differences can be detected between different groups as this is possible on a behavioral level alone.

ERP studies in adult ADHD patients are very sparse. One of the first studies in that field has been published by Duncan et al. [17], describing the ERPs of 13 men with severe developmental dyslexia and 15 normal readers elicited by means of reaction time tasks of varying difficulty presented in the auditory and the visual modality. When tasks were relatively easy, the dyslexic and the healthy group did not differ with regard to the P300 ERP amplitude. In more demanding tasks a difference between the two groups emerged: dyslexic men had reduced amplitude of the visual P300 as compared to the controls. When splitting the dyslexic group in high and low ADHD symptom carriers (during childhood), the authors could show that the persons with many ADHD symptoms were responsible for the differences found on the group level. In contrast, the dyslexic men with no or only few ADHD symptoms during childhood were not different in P300 amplitude from normal readers. In the auditory P300 a hemispheric asymmetry was detected in normal readers with higher amplitudes over the right compared to the left hemisphere. This asymmetry was also found in low-ADHD dyslexics, but not in high-ADHD dyslexics. This loss of a physiological hemispheric asymmetry has been interpreted as pointing to a different brain organization in dyslexic men with an assumed ADHD during childhood.

Fallgatter et al. [18] published another ERP study in adults which considers ADHD symptoms during childhood. The authors investigated prefrontal brain function and cognitive response control in 24 adult patients with personality disorders and ADHD during childhood compared to 12 patients with personality disorders without ADHD during childhood and 24 healthy controls. A visual cued Go/NoGo task (Continuous Performance Test, O/X version) was administered while an ongoing 21-channel EEG was recorded. With topographical analyses the individual NoGo anteriorization (NGA) was assessed. The NGA is the quantitative difference of the centers of gravity of the positive brain electrical field on the anterior posterior axis (centroids) in the P300 time window (measured in electrode positions using a 21-channel array of the extended 10–20 system) during Go trials (Go-centroid) and NoGo trials (NoGo-centroid). In the Go condition the centroid is typically located over parietal brain areas whereas the centroid in the NoGo condition is typically situated over frontocentral brain areas. The NGA is proposed to be a neurophysiologic marker of prefrontal response control. The stability and the short- and long-term test-retest reliability of this measure is excellent [19–22]. The NGA has been shown not to depend on age and gender [23] of the investigated subjects. The LORETA method (low resolution electromagnetic tomography) [24] applied to estimate three-dimensional source localization of ERP data measured at the scalp. This approach revealed that during the NoGo-related anteriorization of the positive electrical field (response inhibition) the activation of the prefrontal cortex (particularly the ACC) is increased compared to Go trials (response execution) [25, 26]. Other brain-imaging methods such as functional magnetic resonance imaging (fMRI) or functional near-infrared spectroscopy (fNIRS) support this finding [27, 28]. The patients with personality disorders and ADHD during childhood showed a significantly reduced mean NGA and diminished amplitudes of the Global Field Power P300 peaks as compared with healthy controls. The increase of frontocentral P300 amplitudes in NoGo-trials was also reduced. Patients with personality disorders alone without ADHD symptomatology during childhood differed from healthy controls in none of these electrophysiological parameters. The authors concluded that their results support the assumption that ADHD-related psychopathology is associated with prefrontal brain dysfunction, which is probably related to processes of response inhibition and/or cognitive response control. Moreover, the three-dimensional source localization analysis with LORETA revealed an electrical dysfunction of the ACC in the NoGo condition in the patients with ADHD symptoms during childhood compared to healthy controls. A corresponding ACC dysfunction has already been found in a sample of boys with ADHD compared to an age-matched control group [29].

In an auditory Go/NoGo task, McPherson and Salamat [30] investigated 11 adults with ADHD (age range 17–25 years) and 20 healthy controls (age range 19–31 years). The research interest was to investigate the effect of variable interstimulus intervals (ISIs, 1, 2, and 4 s) on behavioral reaction time and the auditory P300 ERPs in ADHD. In the auditory task common (1,000, 1,500, and 2,000 Hz) and rare (250 Hz) auditory stimuli were presented. The participants had to ignore the rare (25%) and respond to the frequent stimuli (75%). The authors found that the responses in behavior and electrophysiological parameters were modulated by the different ISIs in the control group, but not in the ADHD group. Parameters that were modulated in the control group were the latency of the P300a and the P300b (increase with increasing ISIs) as well as the amplitude of the P300b (decrease with increasing ISIs), in behavior the number of false alarms and correct rejections (increasing ISI leads to more errors and increased reaction times) were modulated. When the researchers compared the responses of the ADHD and the control adults, the number of hits differed significantly between the two groups for the ISI of 2 s. In all ISIs a significantly different number of false alarms and correct rejections were found for the two groups. ADHD patients were characterized by longer latencies of the P300a and the P300b components in each of the three ISIs. Moreover, ADHD patients displayed lower P3a and P3b amplitudes in the ISIs of 1 and 4 s and the lower P300b amplitudes for the 2 s ISI. The authors interpreted these findings as indications for delayed information processing in ADHD.

The stop signal task is another method to measure inhibitory control which has been proposed to be the core deficit in ADHD [31]. Using such an auditory stop signal task, Bekker et al. [32] investigated 24 adults with ADHD of the combined subtype and the same number of healthy controls. The authors reported the stop signal reaction time to be longer in ADHD adults compared to healthy controls. Nonetheless, no significant differences in the reaction times for Go stimuli were found. In the ADHD patients, lower P3 amplitudes than in healthy controls were detected in stop trials. The authors claimed that the stop P3 reflects inhibitory control. In a dipole source estimation with BESA the generator of the stop P3 was located in the anterior cingulate cortex (ACC). The ACC is presumably related to response inhibition either in a direct way or by a conflict detection system promoting other brain areas to inhibit the action. A similar source location including the ACC has also been found for the NoGo P300 in Go/NoGo tasks [26]. In the same study, another ERP component (N100) generated in the auditory cortex has been investigated, which is presumed to be sensitive to selective attention. Larger N1 amplitudes during successful stops compared to failed stops may reflect increased attention. In line with that assumption, larger N100 components in successful as compared to failed stops were found. However, this difference in N100 amplitude between successful and failed stops was not found in ADHD patients. The authors concluded from these results that disturbed attentional processing of the stop signal contributes to impaired inhibition in adults with ADHD. In healthy controls, better attention reflected in higher N100 amplitudes is associated with a higher probability of correct stopping while in ADHD this association is not existent. This result is in line with the view that failed stopping in healthy controls is related to failed attention *and* failed inhibition, while in ADHD patients failed stopping is only dependent on failed inhibition, as general attention to the stimuli seems not to be affected (i.e. normal reaction time to go stimuli). It could nonetheless be that attention is affected in a way that patients are impaired in the ability to switch their attention to the stop signal. This view would undermine the assumption of response inhibition as a core deficit in ADHD.

As schizophrenia also implies attentional problems including deficits in sensory-gating mechanisms, a deficit in sensory gating can also be expected in ADHD. The P50 double-click paradigm has been established as a neurophysiological measure for sensory-gating mechanisms. The basic observation is that the neuronal activity (P50 component, positive deflection occurring about 50 ms after the click) elicited by an acoustic stimulus (test stimulus) is significantly reduced when it is presented 500 ms after an acoustic stimulus with identical physical properties (conditioning stimulus). Using this electrophysiological approach, Olincy et al. [33] investigated 16 unmedicated ADHD adults, 16 healthy controls and 16 schizophrenic patients. The findings of Olincy et al. [33] did not reveal any differences between the groups in the amplitude of the conditioning P50 response. However, significant differences between the groups were found for the second test stimulus and for the ratio of the test to the conditioning response. These measures were higher in schizophrenic patients as compared to both healthy controls and ADHD patients. The authors concluded that adult patients with ADHD do not have the inhibitory deficits seen in schizophrenia patients. They suggested that the attention problems in both disorders are dependent on different mechanisms. However, a sensory-gating deficit might well be present in a subgroup of ADHD patients, as 25% of the ADHD adults but only 10% of the healthy controls did not suppress the response to the second stimulus in the Olincy et al. study. This possibility should be further investigated in a larger sample of ADHD patients.

Conclusion

There is growing evidence that EEG parameters are impaired in ADHD patients as compared to healthy controls. Moreover, most dysfunctions identified in children with ADHD tend to remain into adulthood, while few parameters are also changing with age. Further investigation is needed, also concerning the question whether there are different subtypes of altered brain function in adult ADHD patients which may serve as endophenotypes. Such putative endophenotypes may be closer related to the genetic variations underlying ADHD than the clinical symptomatology. Finally a better understanding of the pathophysiology underlying ADHD may allow the development of better, individualized treatments.

References

1 Clarke S, Heussler H, Kohn MR: Attention-deficit disorder: not just for children. Intern Med J 2005; 35:721–725.
2 Barry RJ, Clarke AR, Johnstone SJ: A review of electrophysiology in attention-deficit/hyperactivity disorder. I. Qualitative and quantitative electroencephalography. Clin Neurophysiol 2003;114:171–183.
3 Barry RJ, Johnstone SJ, Clarke AR: A review of electrophysiology in attention-deficit/hyperactivity disorder. II. Event-related potentials. Clin Neurophysiol 2003;114:184–198.
4 Brandeis D, van Leeuwen TH, Steger J, Imhof K, Steinhausen HC: Mapping brain functions of ADHD children; in Hirata K, Koga, Y, Nagata K, Yamazaki K (eds): Recent Advances in Human Brain Mapping. Amsterdam, Elsevier, 2002, vol 1232, pp 649–654.
5 Clarke AR, Barry RJ, McCarthy R, Selikowitz M, Croft RJ: EEG differences between good and poor responders to methylphenidate in boys with the inattentive type of attention-deficit/hyperactivity disorder. Clin Neurophysiol 2002;113:1191–1198.
6 Clarke AR, Barry RJ, McCarthy R, Selikowitz M: EEG differences between good and poor responders to methylphenidate and dexamphetamine in children with attention-deficit/hyperactivity disorder. Clin Neurophysiol 2002;113:194–205.
7 Zillessen KE, Scheuerpflug P, Fallgatter AJ, Strik WK, Warnke A: Changes of the brain electrical fields during the continuous performance test in attention-deficit hyperactivity disorder-boys depending on methylphenidate medication. Clin Neurophysiol 2001;112:1166–1173.
8 Seifert J, Scheuerpflug P, Zillessen KE, Fallgatter A, Warnke A: Electrophysiological investigation of the effectiveness of methylphenidate in children with and without ADHD. J Neural Transm 2003;110:821–829.
9 Monastra VJ, Lubar JF, Linden M, et al: Assessing attention-deficit hyperactivity disorder via quantitative electroencephalography: an initial validation study. Neuropsychology 1999;13:424–433.
10 Bresnahan SM, Anderson JW, Barry RJ: Age-related changes in quantitative EEG in attention-deficit/hyperactivity disorder. Biol Psychiatry 1999;46:1690–1697.
11 Bresnahan SM, Barry RJ: Specificity of quantitative EEG analysis in adults with attention-deficit hyperactivity disorder. Psychiatry Res 2002;112:133–144.
12 Bresnahan SM, Barry RJ, Clarke AR, Johnstone SJ: Quantitative EEG analysis in dexamphetamine-responsive adults with attention-deficit/hyperactivity disorder. Psychiatry Res 2006;141:151–159.

13 Hermens DF, Williams LM, Lazzaro I, Whitmont S, Melkonian D, Gordon E: Sex differences in adult ADHD: a double dissociation in brain activity and autonomic arousal. Biol Psychol 2004;66:221–233.
14 Philipsen A, Feige B, Hesslinger B, et al: Sleep in adults with attention-deficit/hyperactivity disorder: a controlled polysomnographic study including spectral analysis of the sleep EEG. Sleep 2005;28: 877–884.
15 Birbaumer N, Schmidt RF: Biologische Psychologie. Heidelberg, Springer, 2006.
16 Picton TW, Bentin S, Berg P, et al: Guidelines for using human event-related potentials to study cognition: recording standards and publication criteria. Psychophysiology 2000;37:127–152.
17 Duncan CC, Rumsey JM, Wilkniss SM, Denckla MB, Hamburger SD, Odou Potkin M: Developmental dyslexia and attention dysfunction in adults: brain potential indices of information processing. Psychophysiology 1994;31:386–401.
18 Fallgatter AJ, Ehlis AC, Rösler M, Strik WK, Blocher D, Herrmann MJ: Diminished prefrontal brain function in adults with psychopathology in childhood related to attention-deficit hyperactivity disorder. Psychiatry Res 2005;138:157–169.
19 Fallgatter AJ, Brandeis D, Strik WK: A robust assessment of the NoGo-anteriorisation of P300 microstates in a cued continuous performance test. Brain Topogr 1997;9:295–302.
20 Bokura H, Yamaguchi S, Kobayashi S: Electrophysiological correlates for response inhibition in a Go/NoGo task. Clin Neurophysiol 2001;112:2224–2232.
21 Fallgatter AJ, Bartsch AJ, Strik WK, et al: Test-retest reliability of electrophysiological parameters related to cognitive motor control. Clin Neurophysiol 2001; 112:198–204.
22 Fallgatter AJ, Aranda DR, Bartsch AJ, Herrmann MJ: Long-term reliability of electrophysiologic response control parameters. J Clin Neurophysiol 2002;19:61–66.
23 Fallgatter AJ, Mueller TJ, Strik WK: Age-related changes in the brain electrical correlates of response control. Clin Neurophysiol 1999;110:833–838.
24 Pascual Marqui RD, Michel CM, Lehmann D: Low resolution electromagnetic tomography: a new method for localizing electrical activity in the brain. Int J Psychophysiol 1994;18:49–65.
25 Strik WK, Fallgatter AJ, Brandeis D, Pascual Marqui RD: Three-dimensional tomography of event-related potentials during response inhibition: evidence for phasic frontal lobe activation. Electroencephalogr Clin Neurophysiol 1998;108:406–413.
26 Fallgatter AJ, Bartsch AJ, Herrmann MJ: Electrophysiological measurements of anterior cingulate function. J Neural Transm 2002;109:977–988.
27 Herrmann MJ, Plichta MM, Ehlis AC, Fallgatter AJ: Optical topography during a Go/NoGo task assessed with multichannel near-infrared spectroscopy. Behav Brain Res 2005;160:135–140.
28 Rubia K, Russell T, Overmeyer S, et al: Mapping motor inhibition: conjunctive brain activations across different versions of go/no-go and stop tasks. Neuroimage 2001;13:250–261.
29 Fallgatter AJ, Ehlis AC, Seifert J, et al: Altered response control and anterior cingulate function in attention-deficit/hyperactivity disorder boys. Clin Neurophysiol 2004;115:973–981.
30 McPherson DL, Salamat MT: Interactions among variables in the P300 response to a continuous performance task in normal and ADHD adults. J Am Acad Audiol 2004;15:666–677.
31 Barkley RA: Behavioral inhibition, sustained attention, and executive functions: constructing a unifying theory of ADHD. Psychol Bull 1997;121:65–94.
32 Bekker EM, Overtoom CC, Kooij JJ, Buitelaar JK, Verbaten MN, Kenemans JL: Disentangling deficits in adults with attention-deficit/hyperactivity disorder. Arch Gen Psychiatry 2005;62:1129–1136.
33 Olincy A, Ross RG, Harris JG, et al: The P50 auditory event-evoked potential in adult attention-deficit disorder: comparison with schizophrenia. Biol Psychiatry 2000;47:969–977.

Prof. Andreas J. Fallgatter, MD
Laboratory for Psychophysiology and Functional Imaging
Department of Psychiatry and Psychotherapy, University Hospital Würzburg
Füchsleinstrasse 15, DE–97080 Würzburg (Germany)
Tel. +49 931 201 77100, Fax +49 931 201 77120, E-Mail Fallgatter_A@klinik.uni-wuerzburg.de

Retz W, Klein RG (eds): Attention-Deficit Hyperactivity Disorder (ADHD) in Adults.
Key Issues in Mental Health. Basel, Karger, 2010, vol 176, pp 88–104

Brain Imaging in Adult Attention-Deficit Hyperactivity Disorder

Marc Schneider[a] · Michael Rösler[b] · Wolfgang Retz[b]

[a]GGZ Noord- en Midden-Limburg, Venray, The Netherlands, and [b]Neurocentre, Saarland University Hospital, Homburg/Saar, Germany

Abstract

This review provides an overview about recent findings in attention-deficit hyperactivity disorder (ADHD) brain imaging. ADHD is understood as a developmental disorder and several studies have addressed brain development in children and adolescents. The hallmarks of impairment of cerebral processing in ADHD are executive dysfunctions (motor execution, inhibitory control, working memory), as well as deficient attention processing. In adulthood, imaging studies have revealed disturbances in the prefrontal cortex, and anterior cingulated cortex (dACC) which are involved in the regulation of selective attention, executive control and decision-making. Dysfunction of basal ganglia is also a consistent finding in ADHD from childhood to adulthood. These findings suggest a persistent dysregulation of frontostriatal circuitries. The cerebellum, and its role in affect and cognition, is also persistently implicated in the pathology of ADHD. The cerebello-(thalamo-)striato-cortical network includes different attention networks and executive control instances. It appears from brain-imaging data in adults that the pathophysiological principles of ADHD do not profoundly change from childhood and adolescence to adulthood, regardless of some changes in psychopathology. The hypothesis of a neurodevelopmental disorder seems to be reinforced on the basis of imaging data of the adults.

Attention-deficit hyperactivity disorder (ADHD) affects adults with a prevalence of about 3–4% [1]. Whereas key symptoms of the psychopathological core symptoms in childhood are inattention, hyperactivity and impulsivity, adults with ADHD tend to be predominantly impaired by attention deficits and disorganization, whereas hyperactivity and impulsivity tend to ameliorate [2, 3]. Emotional dysregulation, mood and anxiety disorders as well as substance abuse are commonly described features and comorbidities in adult patients [4]. As clinical patterns differ between ADHD children and adults, and given that more than half of the children with ADHD do not continue being clinically affected in adulthood, one could hypothesize that adult patients with ADHD represent a distinct subpopulation with distinct neurobiological or environmental background. Therefore, there is a substantial need for neuroanatomical and functional neuroimaging investigations in adults suffering from ADHD. Indeed, like in many areas in neuropsychiatry, neuroimaging techniques have been intensively used also in ADHD research in the past few years.

It is a principle question whether impairment of brain networks compares to those that have been extensively described in ADHD children. Thus, a key question in adult ADHD research is whether there is also impairment of frontostriatal/frontosubcortical networks. These pathways are involved in executive and motor control, as well as in inhibition of behavior and voluntary decision-making. Frontosubcortical networks contain a large amount of noradrenergic, dopaminergic as well as serotonergic projections. Striatal structures, such as putamen, globus pallidum and caudate nucleus, form a frontostriatal network and are typically impaired in ADHD [5]. Areas of particular interest are also the prefrontal and dorsolateral prefrontal cortex (PFC). The anterior cingulated cortex (ACC) seems to play a pivotal role in ADHD psychopathology. This region has widespread connections to forebrain and limbic structures. Besides its function as a conflict monitoring center, the ACC has the role of integrating polymodal inputs from different brain regions in the control of executive and inhibitory functions [6]. Finally, increasing attention is being paid to the cerebellum, which exerts strong influences on affective and cognitive function via thalamic connections [7, 8].

Brain Structure in ADHD

Global Neuroanatomical Findings

Total cerebral volume reduction is well described in children and adolescents with ADHD [9–16], which is most prominent in the right hemisphere. The right hemisphere is hypothesized to play a dominate role in decision-making, inhibitory control and selective attention [17, 18]. It has been shown that damage of the right hemisphere can lead to desynchronization of brain activity and neglect of sensory stimuli [19, 20].

Sowell et al. [21] showed that brain alterations in children with ADHD are focused on those brain regions which are relevant for attention, executive control and linguistic performance. More specifically, they could demonstrate that cortical abnormalities are mainly localized in inferior portions of dorsal PFC and bilateral anterior temporal cortex. Increased gray matter was seen in large portions of the posterior temporal and inferior parietal cortex bilaterally.

Recently, Seidman et al. [22] investigated 24 adults with DSM-IV ADHD and 18 healthy controls comparable on age, socioeconomic status, sex, handedness, education, IQ, and achievement test performance. Compared to controls, adults with ADHD had significantly diminished overall cortical gray matter, and smaller prefrontal and ACC volumes in particular. The authors concluded that adults with ADHD have volume differences in brain regions associated with attention and executive control. These data are largely consistent with studies of children with ADHD, supporting the hypothesis that ADHD is a valid disorder with persistent biological features through all stages of life.

Region-Specific Neuroanatomical Findings

Frontal Lobe

Several studies have confirmed volume reductions of PFC in ADHD children, namely of the dorsolateral part (DLPFC) [9, 10, 13–16, 23]. The DLPFC plays an important role in attention, working memory, planning and organization of a task [18], whereas the ventrolateral prefrontal cortex (VLPFC) is involved in the regulation inhibitory control [24, 25]. The orbitofrontal cortex regulates social behavior and balance of inhibition and desinhibition as well as emotional attribution to decisions.

Hesslinger et al. [26] found diminished left orbitofrontal brain volumes in adult ADHD patients. These regions are associated with social behavior and impulse control. Also in adults with ADHD, selective thinning of cerebral cortex in the networks that subserve attention and executive function was found by Makris et al. [27]. Significant cortical thinning in ADHD was seen especially in the right hemisphere involving the inferior parietal lobule, the dorsolateral prefrontal, and the anterior cingulate cortices. These neuroanatomical data give evidence to the frontal brain abnormalities also in ADHD adults, but the findings need further replication.

Anterior Cingulated Cortex

The dorsal part of the anterior cingulated cortex (dACC) is crucial for executive functioning, inhibitory control monitoring, target detection, error processing as well as reward-based learning. Volume reductions in the right posterior cingulated gyrus in ADHD children have been reported [28]. In adults, lower volumes of the ACC could be shown by in the anatomical study of Makris et al. [27].

Temporal Lobe

Temporal lobes have polymodal sensory integration functions in language comprehension as well as object identification ('what system'), emotional regulation and memory function. The right temporal convexity plays an important role for visuospatial functions, whereas the left temporal convexity contains a large auditory association area which contributes to language comprehension [29]. Sowell et al. [21] demonstrated by anatomical brain surface analysis that children with ADHD had reduced anterior temporal lobe volumes bilaterally. Temporal lobe volume reduction as part of a general brain volume reduction in children and adolescents with ADHD was described by Castellanos et al. [12]. However, there is no substantial information about the interplay between cognition and affect in sensory processing, and its modulation by temporal lobes in ADHD.

Basal Ganglia

The basal ganglia comprise of five nuclei: the caudate nucleus ('cognitive associative' striatum), putamen (sensorimotor striatum), nucleus accumbens (limbic striatum), globus pallidus and subthalamic nucleus. They are closely related to brainstem structures such as substantia nigra and the pedunculopontine nucleus. The striatum comprises the putamen and the pallidum, and displays a high density of dopaminergic neurons. Its main function is procedural learning and automatization of motor programs and behaviors and it serves to assemble complex response habits to strategically adapted environmental needs [30, 31]. ADHD-associated symptoms are associated with striatal damage [32].

Basal ganglia volume reductions have been shown in several studies with ADHD children and adolescents. In most of them uni- or bilateral reduction of caudate volumes were found [9–12, 29, 33–36]. Schrimsher et al. [37] could predict the cumulative severity ratings of inattentive behaviors by measuring caudate volume asymmetry from serial sagittal magnetic resonance images from childhood to adolescence. Also unilateral volume reduction of the pallidum has been shown in several studies in children with ADHD [10–12, 28, 38].

Until now, no evidence for basal ganglia volume reduction in adult ADHD has been reported. A possible explanation is that differences between controls and ADHD almost disappear with increasing age before adulthood [12].

Corpus Callosum

The corpus callosum connects homonymous regions of the cerebral hemispheres. Injury of callosal structures can lead to problems in holding sustained attention [39], with associated deficits in learning and memory [40]. The neuropsychological deficits after injury of corpus callosum are often subtle or lacking.

Volume reduction of the corpus callosum is a common finding in studies with ADHD children and adolescents. Posterior regions of the corpus callosum are mostly affected [15, 41–45]. Data from adult ADHD are lacking so far.

Parietal Lobe

Posner and Petersen [18] have described a posterior attention system located in the parietal lobe, which seems to be mainly modulated by noradrenergic transmission in contrast to the predominantly dopaminergic modulation of the frontal attention system. The posterior part of the parietal cortex is involved in orienting and selective attention networks [46]. It disengages the attentional focus from the contralateral target [47], and lesions of this region can lead to impaired attention [48, 49].

Only few studies have addressed to parietal lobe structure and function in ADHD. Castellanos et al. [12] have shown that posterior parietal volume is reduced, whereas conversely Sowell et al. [21] have demonstrated an increase in cortical volume in children with ADHD. Given its importance in visuospatial orienting and as a region for polymodal sensory integration, it was Makris et al. [27] who pointed out volume reductions in the right inferior parietal lobule in adults with ADHD.

Occipital Lobe

In line with the general findings of Castellanos' work [12], pronounced reduction of left occipital brain volume in children with ADHD was also found by another study group [16]. No data are presently available regarding occipital lobe anatomy in adults with ADHD.

Cerebellum

The role of the cerebellum in cognitive and affective function has been described in 20 patients with cerebellar lesions [50]. Aside from the well-known motor coordination problems, patients with cerebellar lesion display impairment of executive functions, visuospatial cognition deficits as well as blunting of affect and disinhibition of behavior. Cognitive cerebellar functions are located mainly in the posterior lobe (neocerebellum), whereas executive, visuospatial, and memory functions of neocerebellum are impaired when the lesions are located in the hemispheres and dentate nucleus [50, 51]. The vermis has been shown involved with affective disturbances [51]. The cerebellum projects via thalamus to areas in the PFC [52] and there are reciprocal projections from the PFC to cerebellum, thus forming a functional network that influences rather than generates motor control, inhibitory and executive functions. Moreover, several studies have shown that the cerebellum has modulatory effects on forebrain dopamine outflow [53–56].

Several studies in ADHD in childhood and adolescence have shown structural cerebellar impairment [10–12, 15, 16, 57–59]. Indeed, the most marked neuroanatomical anomaly in ADHD has been described in the cerebellum, with volume changes more marked than in the PFC [12]. In children, reductions in right cerebellar hemisphere and vermis volume have been reported [11, 15, 16, 57–59]. These volume reductions correlated with attentional problems and global clinician ADHD ratings [12]. At present there are no data on cerebellar volume in adult ADHD.

Other Brain Regions

In children and adolescents with ADHD an increased volume of the hippocampus bilaterally, which is involved in attentional processes such as visuospatial working memory and executive functions, has been reported [60]. Moreover, some evidence for a reduced size of the basolateral amygdala was found in this study. Since affective symptoms and emotional instability are typical features of and affective disorders are highly prevalent in adult ADHD, altered amygdala and hippocampus volumes are of particular interest also for adults with ADHD. However, in a recent study with adults suffering from ADHD, no differences regarding hippocampus and amygdale volumes were found [61].

Brain Function in ADHD

Functional MRI (fMRI), MRI relaxometry and ligand-bound imaging techniques like SPECT or positron emission tomography (PET) have been used to study functional abnormalities of brain networks in ADHD. From a neurological viewpoint, attention networks can be basically distinguished into three components [18, 46, 62]:

- The arousal and alerting networks are mainly subcortically located and constitute of the ascending reticular activating system. They project to the whole brainstem and thalamus and, through the striatum, up to the limbic system to form cortical projections. The main function of this component is the activation and synchronization of the cerebral cortex during behavior and motivation, and has affinity to salient stimuli and memorization.
- The mixed cortical-subcortical orienting networks are involved in detection of novel stimuli (superior colliculi), filtration of relevant stimuli (pulvinar) and disengagement of attention focus (posterior parietal cortex).
- The selective (or directed/cortical) attentional network is of particular interest for ADHD pathophysiology. It involves frontal brain structures for generation of volitional saccades (frontal eye fields), induces motor intention (premotor cortex), is linked to the working memory (DLPFC) and is modulated by the ACC (target detection, response selection and inhibition, conflict monitoring, motivation) [63]. This network is also called executive (conflict) network and has been shown highly heritable [64]. Within this network, the dACC has strong connectivity to frontal brain structures with dense serotonergic and dopaminergic components. Regions of the parietal cortex also play an important role in mediating sensory functions. The posterior parietal cortex disengages the attentional focus to a target [47] and the superior parietal lobule has the function of voluntary shifts of attention [29]. Right hemisphere dominance could be found for the orienting as well as selective attention [17, 18].

Konrad et al. [65] have used event-related fMRI to investigate brain activations related to these three particular aspects of attention. It could be shown that children with ADHD recruited deviant brain regions for all three above-mentioned attentional networks. ADHD children had less right-sided activation in the anterior cingulated gyrus during alerting, more frontostriatal-insular activation during reorienting, and less frontostriatal activation for executive control. Dysregulation of blood oxygenation level-dependent signals was described in the putamen during reorienting and executive control, suggesting altered strategies in children with ADHD. In medication-naïve children and adolescents with ADHD, task-specific functional abnormalities in frontostriatal but also to parietal and temporal areas were found [66]. Hale et al. [67] concluded from their data that abnormal brain function among adult ADHD participants was not limited to complex executive functions. Abnormal processing of numeric stimuli was indicated during both simple and complex cognitive operations. For example, during the difficult tasks, they exhibited greater activation of left hemispheric linguistic-processing areas and failed to activate bilateral parietal regions important for the complex executive operations.

Anterior Cingulated Cortex

Hypoactivation of the dACC has been consistently described in children and adolescents with ADHD using continuous performance paradigms, with results being similar using fMRI of PET-imaging techniques [25, 68–71]. These findings have led to the hypothesis that dACC plays a significant role in ADHD pathophysiology.

Zametkin et al. [71] were the first to describe hypoactivity of dACC with PET in adult ADHD patients. According to the hypothesis of impairment of selective attention, several studies in adult ADHD have also shown hypofunctionality of the ACC [68, 70]. Following the executive attention hypothesis, the earliest fMRI study in adult ADHD was performed by Bush et al. [70], using a specially designed counting Stroop paradigm. This study demonstrated that the 'cognitive division' of the dACC was not activated in adult ADHD patients during interference conditions. As a compensatory mechanism, ADHD patients activated an alternative frontostriatal network by using different regions of lateral PFC, insular cortex, as well as unilateral activation of caudate, putamen, thalamus and pulvinar. These results may be interpreted as impairment of dACC function in ADHD subjects under conditions where interferences occur, while under conditions where subjects could focus on salient stimuli, there was no difference in dACC activation. This 'normal attention but abnormal stimulus alerting and conflict effect' has also been reported from a neuropsychological point by Oberlin et al. [72]. Only ADHD subjects with the combined type were impaired in their reactions to abrupt visual cues or those that contain conflicting spatial cues. These features were not found in adults with the ADHD-inattentive type.

Besides the role of dACC in selective attentional processing, response selection and inhibition and performance monitoring [73], dACC is also thought to influence reward-based decision-making [74]. The larger the gain, the higher the activity in the pregenual ACC during the decision phase [75]. Ernst et al. [73] found differences in motivational behaviors in ADHD, especially when the patients had to weigh long-term versus short-term rewards. The patients used more parts of the right ACC than healthy controls.

Memory performance was associated with activation of the ACC in healthy adolescents but with activation of the superior parietal lobe (SPL) and precuneus in adolescent ADHD patients [76]. The authors suggested that increased SPL activation in ADHD reflected attentional compensation for low ACC activation during the encoding and that the higher salience of emotional stimuli, in contrast, regulated the interplay between ACC and SPL in conjunction with improving memory to the level of healthy adolescents.

Using a working memory paradigm, Wolf et al. [77] could recently demonstrate lower connectivity in ACC and higher connectivity in dorsal cingulate cortex in adults with ADHD and healthy controls. Another fMRI study found evidence for decreased functional connectivity between ACC and posterior cingulated regions including the precuneus [78].

Motor System

The execution of simple motor tasks reveals distinct cerebral activation pathways. Using a simple finger-tapping task, Mostofsky et al. [79] reported that children with

ADHD had decreased contralateral motor cortex and right parietal cortex activation during right- and left-handed finger sequencing. These findings could be interpreted as anomalous development of cortical systems necessary for execution of patterned movements.

In a study with PET, a correlation between motor hyperactivity with lower binding potential values for dopamine transporter (DAT) in the midbrain was shown in adolescents with ADHD [80]. Thus, altered dopamine signaling might have a causal relationship to hyperactivity. Studies with adult ADHD patients are not available so far.

Frontal Cortex

The most consistent findings in the neuroimaging literature of ADHD are deficits in neural activity within frontostriatal and frontoparietal circuits. However, the results vary across subregions of the frontal cortex, suggesting that ADHD is not associated with dysfunction of any particular part of frontal cortex.

The PFC is critical for the regulation of behavior, attention, and affect by use of representational knowledge. The PFC is important for sustaining attention over a delay, inhibiting distraction, and dividing attention, while more posterior cortical areas are essential for perception and the allocation of attentional resources. The PFC in the right hemisphere is particularly important for behavioral inhibition. Lesions to the PFC produce a profile of distractibility, forgetfulness, impulsivity, poor planning, and locomotor hyperactivity.

Variable findings have been described for VLPFC and DLPFC. These brain regions also monitor attention, planning, working memory and executive control, especially with regard to inhibitory control [18, 81]. Rubia et al. [25] found hypoactivation in the right VLPFC and left caudatus of adolescents with ADHD, whilst Durston et al. [82] reported different activation of frontostriatal regions. Children with ADHD displayed more diffuse network activations including more posterior and dorsolateral prefrontal regions. Rubia et al. [83] reported that medication-naïve adolescent patients with ADHD showed significantly reduced brain activation in the right inferior PFC during successful motor response inhibition and in the precuneus and posterior cingulate gyrus during inhibition failure. These deficits correlated with behavioral scores of ADHD and persisted when corrected for medication history and performance discrepancies. Conversely, Ernst et al. [73] showed using PET that adult ADHD patients, as well as healthy controls, activated VLPFC and DLPFC including insula during a decision-making task. However, the activation of the dACC and hippocampus, subserving emotional and memory processes, was less extended in the ADHD group, who instead recruited the caudal part of the right ACC. These results were interpreted as a basis for problems of motivated behavior in ADHD.

Evidence for significant frontal hypoactivity, including anterior cingulate, dorsolateral prefrontal and inferior prefrontal cortices comes from a meta-analysis of 16 studies with fMRI in children and adolescents with ADHD [84]. Analyses of studies which used other than response inhibition paradigms revealed a more extensive pattern of hypofunction in patients with ADHD than those of response inhibition (thalamus, basal ganglia and parietal cortex). Studies of response inhibition displayed more limited group differences regarding activation of inferior PFC, medial wall regions, and the precentral gyrus.

In adult ADHD patients, less activation and lower functional connectivity was observed during a working memory task in the left VLPC, while connectivity of the right PFC was increased when compared to control subjects together with functional changes in other brain regions [77]. Moreover, a correlation between activation of frontal cortical areas of adult ADHD subjects and inattention scores has been reported, suggesting a functional deficit within this network that depends on the degree of attention deficits [85]. On the other hand, increased activation of orbitofrontal cortex was found in response to gain outcomes during a monetary incentive delay task, suggesting that this part of frontal cortex is involved in abnormal reward processing in adult ADHD [86].

Cerebellum

Due to its involvement in cognitive, emotional processing and behavioral control, the cerebellum seems to be an important region of interest in ADHD research [50]. Anderson et al. [7] reported abnormalities of the vermis in children and adolescents in a MRI relaxometry study that could be influenced by methylphenidate, suggesting an influence of cerebellar function in ADHD. The effects of methylphenidate on cerebellum depended on pretreatment activity level. With fMRI, Schulz et al. [87] described a higher activity of the cerebellum in adolescents with ADHD. In contrast, Valera et al. [88] found significantly decreased activity in cerebellum and also occipital lobe of adult patient with ADHD, even though working memory performance did not differ significantly between ADHD and controls. Kim et al. [89] examined ADHD children with PET and found decreased bilateral cerebellar blood flow in ADHD compared to controls. Volkow et al. [90, 91] reported that methylphenidate could increase metabolic activity of the cerebellum in normal adults, dependent of dopamine receptor activity.

Preliminary results from a study with ADHD children [92] hinted to a relation between cerebellum and forebrain dysfunction and ADHD symptomatology. The authors found with diffusion tensor-imaging technique (DTI) in ADHD prominent white matter abnormalities in the right premotor, right striatal, right cerebral peduncule, left cerebellar peduncule, left cerebellum and left parieto-occipital areas. In adults with ADHD, less activation during a working memory task and changes of functional connectivity of the cerebellum and cortical brain regions was described [77]. These results give additional evidence for corticopontocerebellar circuit deficits in ADHD.

Parietal Cortex

The parietal cortex belongs to an attentional system that includes frontoparietal network structures [18, 93]. For example, orienting networks include the SPL, as well as the temporal parietal junction and frontal eye field [94]. Krauel et al. [76] suggested increased activation in some parietal regions as an attentional compensation for low ACC activation in healthy adolescents. Together with frontal brain areas, the alerting attentional network activates parietal and thalamic areas that are potentially susceptible to the actions of norepinephrine [95–97].

Superior parietal and middle frontal areas are involved in visuospatial processing [98]. Silk et al. [99] have shown in an fMRI study with a mental rotational task, that ADHD children with combined subtype have lower activation of the action-attentional system including superior parietal cortex as well as middle frontal areas. Patients had also increased activation of the posterior midline attentional system. This indicates that ADHD patients might also have parietal dysfunction. As is the case with many of the networks discussed so far, these findings in children have yet to be extended to adults with ADHD. A first step towards this direction has been performed by Tamm et al. [100], who showed that adolescents with ADHD had significant impairments in their ability to direct and allocate attentional resources. This was associated with bilateral aberrations in the parietal attentional system.

Basal Ganglia

In line with PET findings showing reduced basal ganglia perfusion in patients with ADHD [101], subsequent fMRI studies have reported abnormal activation of the striatum [25, 102–104].

Although the main focus of the study of Bush et al. [70] was not the basal ganglia, they observed increased activation of the right putamen in adults with ADHD while performing a Stroop task. Recently, Plichta et al. [105] could show hyporesponsiveness of the ventral-striatal reward system in adults with ADHD, who were examined during a series of choices between two monetary reward options. In addition, they reported increased activation of the dorsal caudate nucleus and amygdala associated with delayed reward. Similarly, decreased activation in the ventral striatum during the anticipation of gain in a monetary incentive delay task was described in another recent study [86]. Moreover, the authors described in this study a negative correlation of ventral striatal activation with self-reported impulsivity and hyperactivity. Similar findings have been reported in a previous fMRI study of brain activation during a reward-anticipation task in adolescents with ADHD [104]. The negative correlation between impulsivity and striatal activation, which was found in both studies, has also been shown by Schneider et al. [85], who used an impulse-control paradigm. Taken together, these results suggest that striatal activation is involved in the processing of reward and the regulation of impulsive-hyperactive traits in adults with ADHD.

ADHD and Comorbid Disorders

Studies with patients who have comorbid disorders or brain lesions are of interest because they may help to validate the specificity of the hypothesized frontostriatal(-cerebellar) dysfunctions and compensatory mechanisms in ADHD.

Bussing et al. [58] have suggested that no differences in cerebellar morphology could be found between ADHD children with and without comorbid conduct disorder. Also, in this study no differences were reported in volume measurements of frontostriatal structures. On the other hand, electrophysiological studies with event-related potentials showed abnormalities in prefrontal lobe activation in teenagers with conduct disorder [106].

Tourette's syndrome (TS) is frequently comorbid with ADHD [107, 108]. In TS, basal ganglia volume reduction and loss of left > right side asymmetry of the globus pallidus is described in some but not all studies [108–110]. Some studies could not differentiate between TS and comorbid ADHD in terms of brain structure alterations, whereas some could find that patients with comorbid ADHD tended to have larger volumes across all cortical portions of those circuits to dorsal prefrontal and parieto-occipital regions and smaller caudate nucleus volumes [111].

Adler et al. [112] have used a simple attention task in adolescents with bipolar disorder and showed that comorbidity with ADHD was associated with less activation of the VLPFC, ACC and higher activation in posterior parietal cortex as well as middle temporal gyrus. Thus, comorbidity with ADHD might result in less activation of prefrontal regions while posterior parietal and temporal cortical areas are used as alternative pathways. Facial recognition is also impaired in ADHD in a similar way when compared with patients with schizophrenia [113]. Both groups display reduced activity in the medial prefrontal and amygdala brain regions required to process emotional faces.

Autism may occur with ADHD and impairment of attention has been consistently reported in autism [114]. In anatomical studies, patients with autism displayed larger total brain and white matter volumes in caudate, globus pallidum, most cortical brain regions and in the cerebellum as compared to ADHD subjects [115]. Reduced fMRI activation was found primarily in amygdala of autistic patients during social tasks [116], but autistic spectrum disorders also display dysfunctional cerebellofrontal spatial attention system [117, 118] similar to ADHD.

Conclusions

In contrast to neuroimaging investigations in children and adolescents with ADHD, the number of studies in adult patients is still limited. Imaging data in general are often confounded by small sample sizes, non-replicated and sometimes even contradictory results. However, recent findings have shown similarities between abnormalities in adult ADHD patients and children with ADHD suggesting impairment of frontostriatal(-cerebellar) networks. Consistent findings have been reported regarding dysfunction of the striatum and the ACC. Prefrontal cortical structures also seem to play a pivotal role in ADHD psychopathology, although these findings are not specific to ADHD. As in children, the cerebellum is also dysfunctional in adults with ADHD. Moreover, there is increasing evidence that also parts of the posterior attention networks are less active in both childhood and adult ADHD. Functional abnormalities comprise frontostriatal, parietal and also temporal cortical areas in a task-specific manner. Attention orienting is less affected than salient stimulus or conflict alerting. Also, several 'vertical' levels of attention networks – beginning from the arousal to the orienting up to the selective attention network – are affected in ADHD.

Data on ADHD patients with comorbid psychiatric disorders are not consistent so far and their contribution to our understanding of ADHD pathophysiology is limited. However, it seems that ADHD symptoms combined with other disorders are associated with frontostriatal dysfunction.

Structural and functional brain-imaging investigations are an important source for our growing knowledge of ADHD pathophysiology. However, due to the lack of sensitivity and specificity of the findings, neuroimaging techniques are not ready to be used as a diagnostic tool. It seems possible that with the progress in understanding the pathogenesis of ADHD together with the technical progress in brain-imaging techniques, we might overcome this shortcoming in future.

References

1 Fayyad J, De Graaf R, Kessler R, Alonso J, Angermeyer M, Demyttenaere K, De Girolamo G, Haro JM, Karam EG, Lara C, Lépine JP, Ormel J, Posada-Villa J, Zaslavsky AM, Jin R: Cross-national prevalence and correlates of adult attention-deficit hyperactivity disorder. Br J Psychiatry 2007;190:402–409.

2 Biederman J, Mick E, Faraone SV: Age-dependent decline of symptoms of attention-deficit hyperactivity disorder: impact of remission definition and symptom type. Am J Psychiatry 2000;157:816–818.

3 Mannuzza S, Klein RG, Bessler A, Malloy P, LaPadula M: Adult outcome of hyperactive boys: educational achievement, occupational rank and psychiatric status. Arch Gen Psychiatry 1993;50:565–576.

4 Retz W, Retz-Junginger P, Hengesch G, Schneider M, Thome J, Pajonk FG, Salahi-Disfan A, Rees O, Wender PH, Rösler M: Psychometric and psychopathological characterization of young male prison inmates with and without attention-deficit/hyperactivity disorder. Eur Arch Psychiatry Clin Neurosci 2004;254:201–208.

5 Casey BJ, Castellanos FX, Giedd JN, Marsh WL, Hamburger SD, Schubert AB, Vauss YC, Vaituzis AC, Dickstein DP, Sarfatti SE, Rapoport JL: Implication of right frontostriatal circuitry in response inhibition and attention-deficit/hyperactivity disorder. J Am Acad Child Adolesc Psychiatry 1997;36:374–383.

6 Carter CS, Macdonald AM, Botvinick M, Ross LL, Stenger VA, Noll D, Cohen JD: Parsing executive processes: strategic vs. evaluative functions of the anterior cingulate cortex. Proc Natl Acad Sci USA 2000;97:1944–1948.

7 Anderson CM, Polcari A, Lowen SB, Renshaw PF, Teicher MH: Effects of methylphenidate on functional magnetic resonance relaxometry of the cerebellar vermis in boys with ADHD. Am J Psychiatry 2002;159:1322–1328.

8 Schmahmann JD: The cerebrocerebellar system: anatomic substrates of the cerebellar contribution to cognition and emotion. Int Rev Psychiatry 2001;13:247–260.

9 Filipek PA, Semrud-Clikeman M, Steingard R, Kennedy D, Biederman J: Volumetric MRI analysis: comparing subjects having attention-deficit hyperactivity disorder with normal controls. Neurology 1997;48:589–601.
10 Castellanos FX, Giedd JN, Marsh WL, Hamburger SD, Vaituzis AC, Dickstein DP, Sarfatti SE, Vauss YC, Snell JW, Lange N, Kaysen D, Krain AL, Ritchie GF, Rajapakse JC, Rapoport JL: Quantitative brain magnetic resonance imaging in attention-deficit hyperactivity disorder. Arch Gen Psychiatry 1996; 53:607–616.
11 Castellanos FX, Giedd JN, Berquin PC, Walter JM, Sharp W, Tran T, Vaituzis AC, Blumenthal JD, Nelson J, Bastain TM, Zijdenbos A, Evans AC, Rapoport JL: Quantitative brain magnetic resonance imaging in girls with attention-deficit/hyperactivity disorder. Arch Gen Psychiatry 2001;58:289–295.
12 Castellanos FX, Lee PP, Sharp W, Jeffries NO, Greenstein DK, Clasen LS, Blumenthal JD, James RS, Ebens CL, Walter JM, Zijdenbos A, Evans AC, Giedd JN, Rapoport JL: Developmental trajectories of brain volume abnormalities in children and adolescents with attention-deficit/hyperactivity disorder. JAMA 2002;288:1740–1748.
13 Kates WR, Frederikse M, Mostofsky SH, Folley BS, Cooper K, Mazur-Hopkins P, Kofman O, Singer HS, Denckla MB, Pearlson GD, Kaufmann WE: MRI parcellation of the frontal lobe in boys with attention-deficit hyperactivity disorder or Tourette syndrome. Psychiatry Res 2002;116:63–81.
14 Mostofsky S, Cooper K, Kates W, Denckla M, Kaufmann W: Smaller prefrontal and premotor volumes in boys with attention-deficit/hyperactivity disorder. Biol Psychiatry 2002;52:785–794.
15 Hill DE, Yeo RA, Campbell RA, Hart B, Vigil J, Brooks W: Magnetic resonance imaging correlates of attention-deficit/hyperactivity disorder in children. Neuropsychology 2003;17:496–506.
16 Durston S, Hulshoff Pol HE, Schnack HG, Buitelaar JK, Steenhuis MP, Minderaa RB, Kahn RS, van Engeland H: Magnetic resonance imaging of boys with attention-deficit/hyperactivity disorder and their unaffected siblings. J Am Acad Child Adolesc Psychiatry 2004;43:332–340.
17 Pardo JV, Pardo P, Janer K, Raichle ME: The anterior cingulated cortex mediates processing selection in the Stroop attention conflict paradigm. Proc Natl Acad Sci USA 1990;87:256–259.
18 Posner MI, Petersen SE: The attention system of the human brain. Annu Rev Neurosci 1990;13:25–42.
19 Heilman KM, Van den Abell T: Right hemisphere dominance for attention: the mechanism underlying hemispheric asymmetries of inattention (neglect). Neurology 1980;30:327–330.
20 Weintraub S, Mesulam MM: Right cerebral dominance in spatial attention: further evidence based on ipsilateral neglect. Arch Neurol 1987;44:621–625.
21 Sowell ER, Thompson PM, Welcome SE, Henkenius AL, Toga AW, Peteron BS: Cortical abnormalities in children and adolescents with attention-deficit hyperactivity disorder. Lancet 2003;362:1699–1707.
22 Seidman LJ, Valera EM, Makris N, Monuteaux MC, Boriel DL, Kelkar K, Kennedy DN, Caviness VS, Bush G, Aleardi M, Faraone SV, Biederman J: Dorsolateral prefrontal and anterior cingulate cortex volumetric abnormalities in adults with attention-deficit/hyperactivity disorder identified by magnetic resonance imaging. Biol Psychiatry 2006; 60:1071–1080.
23 Hynd GW, Semrud-Clikeman MS, Lorys AR, Novey ES, Eliopulos D: Brain morphology in developmental dyslexia and attention-deficit/hyperactivity. Arch Neurol 1990;47:919–926.
24 Aron AR, Fletcher PC, Bullmore ET, Sahakian BJ, Robbins TW: Stop-signal inhibition disrupted by damage to the right inferior frontal gyrus in humans. Nat Neurosci 2003;6:115–116.
25 Rubia K, Overmeyer S, Taylor E, Brammer M, Williams SC, Simmons A, Bullmore ET: Hypofrontality in attention-deficit hyperactivity disorder during higher-order motor control: a study with functional MRI. Am J Psychiatry 1999;156:891–896.
26 Hesslinger B, Tebartz van Elst L, Thiel T, Haegele K, Hennig J, Ebert D: Frontoorbital volume reductions in adult patients with attention-deficit hyperactivity disorder. Neurosci Lett 2002;328:319–321.
27 Makris N, Biederman J, Valera EM, Bush G, Kaiser J, Kennedy DN, Caviness VS, Faraone SV, Seidman LJ: Cortical thinning of the attention and executive function networks in adults with attention-deficit/ hyperactivity disorder. Cereb Cortex 2007;17:1364–1375.
28 Overmeyer S, Bullmore ET, Suckling J, Simmons A, Williams SC, Santosh PJ, Taylor E: Distributed grey and white matter deficits in hyperkinetic disorder: MRI evidence for anatomical abnormality in an attentional network. Psychol Med 2001;31:1425–1435.
29 Devinski O, D'Esposito M: Neurology of cognitive and behavioral disorders; in Contemporary Neurology Series 68. London, Oxford University Press, 2004, pp 103–121.
30 Marsden CD: Functions of the basal ganglia. Rinsho Shinkeigaku 1982;22:1093–1094.
31 Dubois D, Defontaines B, Deweer B, Malapani C, Pillon B: Cognitive and behavioural changes in patients with focal lesions of the basal ganglia. Adv Neurol 1995;65:29–41.

32 Lou H: Etiology and pathogenesis of attention-deficit hyperactivity disorder; significance of prematurity and perinatal hypoxic-haemodynamic encephalopathy. Acta Paediatr 1996;85:1266–1271.
33 Castellanos FX, Giedd JN, Eckburg P, Marsh WL, Vaituzis AC, Kaysen D, Hamburger SD, Rapoport JL: Quantitative morphology of the caudate nucleus in attention-deficit hyperactivity disorder. Am J Psychiatry 1994;151:1791–1796.
34 Castellanos FX, Sharp WS, Gottesman RF, Greenstein DK, Giedd JN, Rapoport JL: Anatomic brain abnormalities in monozygotic twins discordant for attention-deficit disorder. Am J Psychiatry 2003;160: 1693–1696.
35 Hynd GW, Hern KL, Novey ES, Eliopulos D, Marshall R, Gonzalez JJ, Voeller KK: Attention deficit-hyperactivity disorder and asymmetry of the caudate nucleus. J Child Neurol 1993;8:339–347.
36 Mataro M, Garcia-Sanchez C, Junque C, Estevez-Gonzalez A, Pujol J: Magnetic resonance imaging measurement of the caudate nucleus in adolescents with attention-deficit hyperactivity disorder and its relationship with neuropsychological and behavioral measures. Arch Neurol 1997;54:963–968.
37 Schrimsher GW, Billingsley RL, Jackson EF, Moore BD 3rd: Caudate nucleus volume asymmetry predicts attention-deficit hyperactivity disorder symptomatology in children. J Child Neurol 2002;17: 877–884.
38 Aylward EH, Reiss AL, Reader MJ, Singer HS, Brown JE, Denckla MB: Basal ganglia volumes in children with attention-deficit hyperactivity disorder. J Child Neurol 1996;11:112–115.
39 Ellenberg L, Sperry RW: Capacity for holding sustained attention following comissurotomy. Cortex 1979;15:421–438.
40 Zaidel DW: Memory and spatial cognition following commissurotomy; in Boller F, Grafman J (eds): Handbook of Neuropsychology. Amsterdam, Elsevier, 1990
41 Baumgardner TL, Singer HS, Denckla MB, Rubin MA, Abrams MT, Colli MJ, Reiss AL: Corpus callosum morphology in children with Tourette syndrome and attention-deficit hyperactivity disorder. Neurology 1996;47:1–6.
42 Giedd JN, Castellanos FX, Casey BJ, Kozuch P, King AC, Hamburger SD, Rapoport JL: Quantitative morphology of the corpus callosum in attention-deficit hyperactivity disorder. Am J Psychiatry 1994;151:665–669.
43 Hynd GW, Semrud-Clikeman M, Lorys AR, Novey ES, Eliopulos D, Lytinen H: Corpus callosum morphology in attention-deficit hyperactivity disorder: morphometric analysis of MRI. J Learn Disabil 1991;24:141–146.
44 Lyoo I, Noam G, Lee C, Lee H, Kennedy B, Renshaw P: The corpus callosum and lateral ventricles in children with attention-deficit hyperactivity disorder: a brain magnetic resonance imaging study. Biol Psychiatry 1996;40:1060–1063.
45 Semrud-Clikeman MS, Filipek PA, Biederman J, Steingard R, Kennedy D, Renshaw P, Bekken K: Attention-deficit hyperactivity disorder: Magnetic resonance imaging morphometric analysis of the corpus callosum. J Am Acad Child Adolesc Psychiatry 1994;33:875–881.
46 Fan J, Bruce T, McCandliss D, Fossella J, Flombaum J, Posner MI: The activation of attentional networks. Neuroimage 2005;26:471–479.
47 Rafal R, Robertson L: The neurology of visual attention; in Gazzaniga MS (ed): The Cognitive Neurosciences. Cambridge/MA, MIT Press, 1995, pp 625–648.
48 Posner MI: Attention in cognitive neuroscience: an overview; in Gazzaniga MS (ed): The Cognitive Neurosciences. Cambridge/MA, MIT Press, 1995, pp 615–624.
49 Ro T, Borden C, Driver J, Rafal R: Ipsilesional biases in saccades but not perception after lesions of the human inferior parietal lobule. J Cogn Neurosci 2001;13:920–929.
50 Schmahmann JD, Sherman JC: The cerebellar cognitive affective syndrome. Brain 1998;121:561–579.
51 Schmahmann JD: Disorders of the cerebellum: ataxia, dysmetria of thought, and the cerebellar cognitive affective syndrome. J Neuropsychiatry Clin Neurosci 2004;16:367–378.
52 Middleton FA, Strick PL: Cerebellar projections to the prefrontal cortex of the primate. J Neurosci 2001;21:700–712.
53 Snider SR, Snider RS: Structural and functional relationships between cerebellum and catecholamine systems: an overview. Exp Brain Res Suppl 1982;6: 557–606.
54 Tellerman K, Astrow A, Fahn S, Snider SR, Snider RS, Glassgold JM: Cerebellar control of catecholaminergic activities: implications for drug therapy of movement disorders. Int J Neurol 1979;13: 135–155.
55 Glowinski J, Nieoullon A, Cheramy A: Regulations of the activity of the nigrostriatal dopaminergic pathways by cortical, cerebellar, and sensory neuronal afferences. Adv Biochem Psychopharmacol 1978;19:75–87.
56 Nieoullon A, Cheramy A, Glowinski J: Control of the activity of the two dopaminergic systems by cortical, cerebellar and sensory afferents in the cat. Appl Neurophysiol 1979;42:51–53.

57 Berquin PC, Giedd JN, Jacobsen LK, Hamburger SD, Krain AL, Rapoport JL, Castellanos FX: Cerebellum in attention-deficit hyperactivity disorder: a morphometric MRI study. Neurology 1998; 50:1087–1093.
58 Bussing R, Grudnik J, Mason D, Wasiak M, Leonard C: ADHD and conduct disorder: an MRI study in a community sample. World J Biol Psychiatry 2002; 3:216–220.
59 Mostofsky SH, Reiss AL, Lockhart P, Denckla MB: Evaluation of cerebellar size in attention-deficit hyperactivity disorder. J Child Neurol 1998;13:434–439.
60 Plessen KJ, Bansal R, Zhu H, Whiteman R, Amat J, Quackenbush GA, Martin L, Durkin K, Blair C, Royal J, Hugdahl K, Peterson BS: Hippocampus and amygdala morphology in attention-deficit/hyperactivity disorder. Arch Gen Psychiatry 2006;63:795–807.
61 Perlov E, Philipsen A, Tebartz van Elst L, Ebert D, Henning J, Maier S, Bubl E, Hesslinger B: Hippocampus and amygdala morphology in adults with attention-deficit hyperactivity disorder. J Psychiatry Neurosci 2008;33:509–515.
62 Coull JT, Frith CD, Frackowiak RS, Grasby PM: A fronto-parietal network for rapid visual information processing: a PET study of sustained attention and working memory. Neuropsychologia 1996;34:1085–1095.
63 Bush G, Luu P, Posner MI: Cognitive and emotional influences in anterior cingulate cortex. Trends Cogn Sci 2000:4:215–222.
64 Fan J, Wu Y, Fossella JA, Posner MI: Assessing the heritability of attentional networks. BMC Neurosci 2001;2:14.
65 Konrad K, Neufang S, Hanisch C, Fink GR, Herpertz-Dahlmann B: Dysfunctional attentional networks in children with attention-deficit/hyperactivity disorder: evidence from an event-related functional magnetic resonance imaging study. Biol Psychiatry 2006;59:643–651.
66 Smith AB, Taylor E, Brammer M, Tone B, Rubia K: Task-specific hypoactivation in prefrontal and temporoparietal brain regions during motor inhibition and task switching in medication-naïve children and adolescents with attention-deficit hyperactivity disorder. Am J Psychiatry 2006;163:1044–1051.
67 Hale TS, Bookheimer S, McGough JJ, Phillips JM, McCracken JT: Atypical brain activation during simple and complex levels of processing in adult ADHD: an fMRI study. J Atten Disord 2007;11:125–140.
68 Durston S: A review of the biological bases of ADHD: What have we learned from imaging studies? Ment Retard Dev Disabil Res Rev 2003;9:184–195.
69 Tamm L, Menon V, Ringel J, Reiss A: Event-related fMRI evidence of frontotemporal involvement in aberrant response inhibition and task switching in attention-deficit/hyperactivity disorder. J Am Acad Child Adolesc Psychiatry 2004;43:1430–1440.
70 Bush G, Frazier JA, Rauch SL, Seidman LJ, Whalen PJ, Jenike MA, Rosen BR, Biederman J: Anterior cingulate cortex dysfunction in attention-deficit/hyperactivity disorder revealed by fMRI and the counting Stroop. Biol Psychiatry 1999;45:1542–1552.
71 Zametkin AJ, Nordahl TE, Gross M, King AC, Semple WE, Rumsey J, Hamburger S, Cohen RM: Cerebral glucose metabolism in adults with hyperactivity of childhood onset. N Engl J Med 1990;323: 1361–1366.
72 Oberlin BG, Alford JL, Marrocco RT: Normal attention but abnormal stimulus alerting and conflict effect in combined subtype of ADHD. Behav Brain Res 2005;165:1–11.
73 Ernst M, Kimes AS, London ED, Matochik JA, Eldreth D, Tata S, Contoreggi C, Leff M, Bolla K: Neural substrates of decision-making in adults with attention-deficit hyperactivity disorder. Am J Psychiatry 2003;160:1061–1070.
74 Bush G, Vogt BA, Holmes J, Dale AM, Greve D, Jenike MA, Rosen BR: Dorsal anterior cingulate cortex: a role in reward-based decision-making. Proc Natl Acad Sci USA 2002;99:523–528.
75 Rogers RD, Ramnani N, Mackay C, Wilson JL, Jezzard P, Carter CS, Smith SM: Distinct portions of anterior cingulated cortex and medial prefrontal cortex are activated by reward processing in separable phases of decision-making cognition. Biol Psychiatry 2004;55:594–602.
76 Krauel K, Duzel E, Hinrichs H, Santel S, Rellum T, Baving L: Impact of emotional salience on episodic memory in attention-deficit/hyperactivity disorder: a functional magnetic resonance imaging study. Biol Psychiatry 2007;61:1370–1379.
77 Wolf RC, Plichta MM, Sambataro F, Fallgatter AJ, Jacob C, Lesch KP, Herrmann MJ, Schönfeldt-Lecuona C, Connemann BJ, Grön G, Vasic N: Regional brain activation changes and abnormal functional connectivity of the ventrolateral prefrontal cortex during working memory processing in adults with attention-deficit/hyperactivity disorder. Human Brain Mapp 2008; in press.
78 Castellanos FX, Margulies DS, Kelly C, Uddin LQ, Ghaffari M, Kirsch A, Shaw D, Shezad Z, Di Martino A, Biswal B, Sonuga-Barke EJ, Rotrosen J, Adler LA, Milham MP: Cingulate-precuneus interactions: a new locus of dysfunction in adult attention-deficit/hyperactivity disorder. Biol Psychiatry 2008;63:332–337.

79 Mostofsky SH, Rimrodt SL, Schafer JG, Boyce A, Goldberg MC, Pekar JJ, Denckla MB: Atypical motor and sensory cortex activation in attention-deficit/hyperactivity disorder: a functional magnetic resonance imaging study of simple sequential finger tapping. Biol Psychiatry 2006;59:48–56.
80 Jucaite A, Fernell E, Halldin C, Forssberg H, Farde L: Reduced midbrain dopamine transporter binding in male adolescents with attention-deficit/hyperactivity disorder: association between striatal dopamine markers and motor hyperactivity. Biol Psychiatry 2005;57:229–238.
81 Duncan J, Owen AM: Common regions of the human frontal lobe recruited by diverse cognitive demands. Trends Neurosci 2000;23:475–483.
82 Durston S, Tottenham NT, Thomas KM, Davidson MC, Eigsti IM, Yang Y, Ulug AM, Casey BJ: Differential patterns of striatal activation in young children with and without ADHD. Biol Psychiatry 2003;53:871–878.
83 Rubia K, Smith AB, Brammer MJ, Toone B, Taylor E: Abnormal brain activation during inhibition and error detection in medication-naive adolescents with ADHD. Am J Psychiatry 2005;162:1067–1075.
84 Dickstein SG, Bannon K, Xavier Castellanos F, Milham MP: The neural correlates of attention-deficit hyperactivity disorder: an ALE meta-analysis. J Child Psychol Psychiatry 2006;47:1051–1062.
85 Schneider M, Krick C, Retz W, Hengesch G, Retz-Junginger P, Reith W, Rösler M: Impairment of fronto-striatal and parietal cerebral networks correlates with attention-deficit hyperactivity disorder psychopathology in adults – a functional magnetic resonance imaging study. Psychiatry Res Neuroimaging 2009 (submitted).
86 Ströhle A, Stoy M, Wrase J, Schwarzer S, Schlangenhauf F, Huss M, Hein J, Nedderhut A, Neumann B, Gregor A, Juckel G, Knutson B, Lehmkuhl U, Bauer M, Heinz A: Reward anticipation and outcomes in adult males with attention-deficit/hyperactivity disorder. Neuroimage 2008;39:966–972.
87 Schulz KP, Fan J, Tang CY, Newcorn JH, Buchsbaum MS, Cheung AM, Halperin JM: Response inhibition in adolescents diagnosed with attention-deficit hyperactivity disorder during childhood: an event-related FMRI study. Am J Psychiatry 2004;161:1650–1657.
88 Valera EM, Faraone SV, Biederman J, Poldrack RA, Seidman LJ: Functional neuroanatomy of working memory in adults with attention-deficit/hyperactivity disorder. Biol Psychiatry 2005;57:439–447.
89 Kim BN, Lee JS, Shin MS, Cho SC, Lee DS: Regional cerebral perfusion abnormalities in attention-deficit/hyperactivity disorder. Statistical parametric mapping analysis. Eur Arch Psychiatry Clin Neurosci 2002;252:219–225.
90 Volkow ND, Wang G-J, Fowler JS, Logan J, Angriest B, Hitzemann R, Lieberman J, Pappas N: Effects of methylphenidate on regional brain glucose metabolism in humans: relationship to dopamine D2 receptors. Am J Psychiatry 1997;154:50–55.
91 Volkow ND, Wang GJ, Fowler JS, Hitzemann R, Gatley J, Ding YS, Wong C, Pappas N: Differences in regional brain metabolic responses between single and repeated doses of methylphenidate. Psychiatry Res 1998;83:29–36.
92 Ashtari M, Kumra S, Bhaskar SL, Clarke T, Thaden E, Cervellione KL, Rhinewine J, Kane JM, Adesman A, Milanaik R, Maytal J, Diamond A, Szeszko P, Ardekani BA: Attention-deficit/hyperactivity disorder: a preliminary diffusion tensor imaging study. Biol Psychiatry 2005;57:448–455.
93 Mesulam MM: Large-scale neurocognitive networks and distributed processing for attention, language and memory. Ann Neurol 1990;28:597–613.
94 Corbetta M, Shulman GL: Control of goal-directed and stimulus-driven attention in the brain. Nat Rev Neurosci 2002;3:201–215.
95 Coull JT, Buchel C, Friston KJ, Frith CD: Noradrenergically mediated plasticity in a human attentional neuronal network. Neuroimage 1999;10:705–715.
96 Coull JT, Frith CD, Buchel C, Nobre AC: Orienting attention in time: behavioural and neuroanatomical distinction between exogenous and endogenous shifts. Neuropsychologia 2000;38:808–819.
97 Coull JT, Nobre AC, Frith CD: The noradrenergic α_2-agonist clonidine modulates behavioural and neuroanatomical correlates of human attentional orienting and alerting. Cereb Cortex 2001;11:73–84.
98 Booth JR, Burman DD, Meyer JR, Lei Z, Trommer BL, Davenport ND, Li W, Parrish TB, Gitelman DR, Mesulam MM: Larger deficits in brain networks for response inhibition than for visual selective attention in attention-deficit hyperactivity disorder. J Child Psychol Psychiatry 2005;46:94–111.
99 Silk T, Vance A, Rinehart N, Egan G, O'Boyle M, Bradshaw JL, Cunnington R: Fronto-parietal activation in attention-deficit hyperactivity disorder, combined type: functional magnetic resonance imaging study. Br J Psychiatry 2005;187:282–283.
100 Tamm L, Menon V, Reiss AL: Parietal attentional system aberrations during target detection in adolescents with attention-deficit hyperactivity disorder: event-related fMRI evidence Am J Psychiatry 2006;163:1033–1043.
101 Lou HC, Henriksen L, Bruhn P, Børner H, Nielsen JB: Striatal dysfunction in attention-deficit and hyperkinetic disorder. Arch Neurol 1989;46:48–52.

102 Teicher MH, Anderson CM, Polcari A, Glod CA, Maas LC, Renshaw PF: Functional deficits in basal ganglia of children with attention-deficit/hyperactivity disorder shown with functional magnetic resonance imaging relaxometry. Nat Med 2000;6: 470–473.

103 Vaidya CJ, Austin G, Kirkorian G, Ridlehuber HW, Desmond JE, Glover GH, Gabrieli JD: Selective effects of methylphenidate in attention-deficit hyperactivity disorder: a functional magnetic resonance study. Proc Natl Acad Sci USA 1998;95:14494–14499.

104 Scheres A, Milham MP, Knutson B, Castellanos FX: Ventral striatal hyporesponsiveness during reward anticipation in attention-deficit/hyperactivity disorder. Biol Psychiatry 2007;61:720–724.

105 Plichta MM, Vasic N, Wolf RC, Lesch KP, Brummer D, Jacob C, Fallgatter AJ, Grön G: Neural hyporesponsiveness and hyperresponsiveness during immediate and delayed reward processing in adult attention-deficit/hyperactivity disorder. Biol Psychiatry 2009;65:7–14.

106 Bauer LO, Hesselbrock VM: Brain maturation and subtypes of conduct disorder: interactive effects on p300 amplitude and topography in male adolescents. J Am Acad Child Adolesc Psychiatry 2003; 42:106–115.

107 Comings DE, Comings BG: Tourette syndrome clinical and psychological aspects of 250 cases. Am J Hum Genet 1985;37:435–450.

108 Spencer T, Biedermann J, Harding M, Hallett JJ, Laurino JP, Benson M, Kiessling LS: The relationship between tic disorders and Tourette's syndrome revisited. J Am Acad Child Adolesc Psychiatry 1995; 34:1133–1139.

109 Peterson B, Riddle MA, Cohen DJ, Katz LD, Smith JC, Hardin MT, Leckman JF: Reduced basal ganglia volumes in Tourette's syndrome using three-dimensional reconstruction techniques from magnetic resonance images. Neurology 1993;43:941–949.

110 Singer HS: Neurobiology of Tourette syndrome. Neurol Clin North Am 1997;15:357–378.

111 Peterson BS: Neuroimaging studies of Tourette syndrome: a decade of progress. Adv Neurol 2001;85: 179–196.

112 Adler CM, Delbello MP, Mills NP, Schmithorst V, Holland S, Strakowski SM: Comorbid ADHD is associated with altered patterns of neuronal activation in adolescents with bipolar disorder performing a simple attention task. Bipolar Disord Dec 2005;7:577–588.

113 Marsh PJ, Williams LM: ADHD and schizophrenia phenomenology: visual scanpaths to emotional faces as a potential psychophysiological marker? Neurosci Biobehav Rev 2006;30:651–656.

114 Allen G, Courchesne E: Attention function and dysfunction in autism. Front Biosci 2001;6:D105–D119.

115 Piven J, Arndt S, Bailey J, Andreasen N: Regional brain enlargement in autism: a magnetic resonance imaging study. J Am Acad Child Adolesc Psychiatry 1996;35:530–536.

116 Baron-Cohen S, Ring HA, Wheelwright S, Bullmore ET, Brammer MJ, Simmons A, Williams SC: Social intelligence in the normal and autistic brain: an fMRI study. Eur J Neurosci 1999;11:1891–1898.

117 Allen G, Muller RA, Courchesne E: Cerebellar function in autism: functional magnetic resonance image activation during a simple motor task. Biol Psychiatry 2004;56:269–278.

118 Haist F, Adamo M, Westerfield M, Courchesne E, Townsend J: The functional neuroanatomy of spatial attention in autism spectrum disorder. Dev Neuropsychol 2005;27:425–458.

Dr. Marc Schneider, MD
GGZ Noord- en Midden-Limburg
NL–5803 AC Venray (The Netherlands)
Tel. +31 478 527527, Fax +31 478 527057, E-Mail MSchneider@ggznml.nl

Retz W, Klein RG (eds): Attention-Deficit Hyperactivity Disorder (ADHD) in Adults.
Key Issues in Mental Health. Basel, Karger, 2010, vol 176, pp 105–125

Attention-Deficit Hyperactivity Disorder in Adults: Diagnosis and Prevalence

Rolf-Dieter Stieglitz

University Hospital Basel, Basel, Switzerland

Abstract

Attention-deficit hyperactivity disorder (ADHD) is meanwhile accepted as a valid diagnostic entity in adults. A comprehensive and thorough examination, using a multimodel approach, is essential to diagnose ADHD in adults. Several diagnostic instruments exist which serve as important building blocks for a reliable ADHD diagnosis. Because the ADHD diagnosis is ultimately a clinical diagnosis, assessment instruments fulfill an important function in addition to other aspects, e.g. medical history. To diagnose ADHD in a reliable manner is important for clinical practice as well as for research, especially for the estimation of prevalence rates.

Introduction

In the field of attention-deficit hyperactivity disorder (ADHD) in adulthood, two subject areas are of particular significance, and both are similarly difficult to observe. These are, on the one hand, estimation of the prevalence of the disorder, and on the other hand the diagnostic procedures. Both are closely linked and should therefore be dealt with together. With regard to prevalence, the problem still persists that only unsatisfactory data are available, or rather only approximate estimates. This is accompanied in turn with diagnostic problems. ADHD is not usually included in the large international epidemiological studies. This is because the instruments used (see below) only include the disorders in adulthood, and they do not allow for other disorders to be considered. The reason for this is that, until a few years ago, the view was that ADHD would not even exist in adulthood. It is only gradually becoming accepted that this is not the case, by means of heightened efforts, on the one hand, to provide reliable estimates of the prevalence of the disorder also in adulthood as well as, on the other hand, to develop appropriate instruments which allow reliable assessment. Several developments have been observed here over recent years. Diagnosis today (at least in research) is usually based on the criteria of the Diagnostic and Statistical

Manual of Mental Disorders, Fourth Edition (DSM-IV [1]) in clinical practice it is often made following the International Classification of Diseases, Tenth Revision (ICD-10 [2]). Both definitions are similar, though not identical. Table 1 contains the main characteristics of both definitions of the disorder. The main difference between both systems are the number of (sub)types of ADHD which can be diagnosed. The DSM-IV defines three main subtypes and two additional subtypes, ICD-10 only one main subtype and two additional subtypes.

A reliable diagnosis is the precondition for an appropriate therapy which is of particular importance in ADHD [see 3]. Following a successful diagnosis, it is necessary to document the course of treatment, for which, again, diagnostic instruments in the form of rating scales or interviews are necessary. The objective of this paper is to give a current overview of diagnostic procedures as well as prevalence rates of the disorder.

General Problems in the Assessment of ADHD in Adults

Diagnosis of ADHD in adults is characterized, in contrast to the diagnosis of other psychiatric disorders, by a range of particular features which will now be briefly detailed.

Patient. The central data source is usually the patient. General conditions for the assessment of psychological phenomena must be considered here: cognitive factors such as intelligence, language comprehension, ability for introspection and ability to remember as well as non-cognitive factors such as motivation and readiness to give information about oneself. One particular aspect is worth mentioning. Because ADHD is a disorder which begins very early, and is, moreover, continually present, patients often have the impression that certain symptoms are a part of their life and are not necessarily a component of a disorder. The patient knows himself just as he is. The symptoms of inattention, impulsivity and hyperactivity develop not just after more or less normal development as the result of an illness, but rather exist from the beginning on. The patient, following his experience, has therefore no reason to feel 'ill'. It is often only in comparison to people not affected (by ADHD) or when experiencing increasing problems in coping with life that the problems become clear.

The diagnosis of ADHD in adulthood is based, along with symptomatology, essentially on assessment of functional impairment in childhood, rarely on objective reports from the past (e.g. school reports). Retrospective statements are therefore of central significance, although prone to inaccuracy, incompleteness or other distortions. This is of significance then, as most patients who undergo an assessment were not assessed in childhood or adolescence.

Rater. As in other psychiatric disorders the independent rater represents a further important data source. It is, however, a problem that symptoms are often difficult or impossible to observe in the examination situation. Symptomatology is more likely to be reported from patients than observed. Adults do not jump around during the

Table 1. Diagnostic criteria for ADHD: DSM-IV [1] and ICD-10 research criteria [2]

	DSM-IV	ICD-10
Symptom criteria	*Two domains:* – *Inattention:* 9 symptoms (e.g. difficulty organizing tasks and activities, easily distracted by extraneous stimuli); 6 or more symptoms necessary (criterion A1) – *Hyperactivity-impulsivity:* 9 symptoms (e.g. hyperactivity, 6 symptoms: e.g. talks excessively; impulsivity: 3 symptoms: e.g. difficulty awaiting turn); 6 or more symptoms necessary (criterion A2)	*Three domains:* – *Attention:* 9 symptoms (e.g. often impaired in organizing tasks and activities; often fails to sustain attention in tasks); 6 or more symptoms necessary – *Hyperactivity:* 5 symptoms (e.g. often fidgets with hands or feet or squirms on seat; exhibits a persistent pattern of excessive motor activity); 3 or more symptoms necessary – *Impulsivity:* 4 symptoms (e.g. often blurts out answers before questions have been completed; often fails to wait in lines…), 1 or more symptoms necessary
Onset and duration	Before age 7 years; at least 6 months	Before age 7 years; at least 6 months
Impairments	In two or more settings (e.g. at school/work or at home) Clinically significant impairment in social, academic, or occupational functioning	Clinically significant distress or impairment in social, academic, or occupational functioning
Exclusion criteria	Symptoms do not occur exclusively during the course of other psychiatric disorders (e.g. schizophrenia) or not better accounted for by another mental disorder (e.g. mood disorder)	Several other psychiatric disorders (e.g. mood disorder, anxiety disorder)
Diagnostic algorithm and diagnosis	Attention-deficit hyperactivity disorders, combined type (criteria A1 and A2) attention-deficit hyperactivity disorders, predominantly inattentive type (criterion A1) Attention-deficit hyperactivity disorders, predominantly hyperactive-impulsive type (criterion A2) 314.9 Attention-deficit hyperactivity disorders, disorder not otherwise specified	F90 Hyperkinetic disorders F90.0 Disturbance of activity and attention F90.1 Hyperkinetic conduct disorder F90.8 Other hyperkinetic disorder
Comments	'In partial remission': symptoms are present, but not full criteria	No subtypes available

assessment like children and do not hop from chair to chair. What is directly observable in adults is a rather unobtrusive motor restlessness or lack of concentration. Many other symptoms elude direct examination (e.g. intrapsychic phenomena such as inner tension, restlessness). In the evaluation assessment of these phenomena, the diagnostician is therefore reliant on statements from significant others and from the patient himself.

Assessment Instruments. Although ADHD is just a relatively 'young' disorder in the adult domain, several instruments with a different focus already exist (see below). Many instruments are based on the DSM-IV criteria. Problems often occur in the appropriate conversion of these criteria to statements for the adult domain. Moreover, as yet, no diagnostic standard exists and in many cases, there are no authorized translations in other languages and even fewer systematic validity studies.

Classification System. Both current classification systems do not accord in the operationalization of the disorder. The threshold for the disorder, to name one aspect, is higher in ICD-10 because there is only one type, whereas in DSM-IV there are different subtypes (see table 1). However, neither system has particular criteria for adults. Furthermore, the diagnostic criteria are not exclusive for an ADHD, but rather exhibit the following problems: (1) the majority are non-specific (e.g. attention) and (2) they show overlap to other psychiatric disorders (e.g. borderline personality disorder, see below).

As well as the problematic transfer of criteria to adults, there is also the question of how practical and valid the age-at-onset criterion of 7 years is [see 10].

Conceptualization of the Disorder. Closely linked to questions of classification is the question of whether the disorder should be seen as dimensional or categorical [see in general 11]. This issue often discussed in the context of many psychiatric disorders (e.g. personality disorders) is also discussed in ADHD [see e.g. 12]. ADHD can be regarded as a dimensional construct. It is not a matter of an all-or-nothing principle. ADHD represents rather the end of a continuum of a normal distribution. A combination of the categorical point of view and a dimensional perspective seems therefore appropriate. Moreover, the core symptoms of the disorder are, similarly, general characteristics of human nature such as e.g. inattention or impulsivity, particularly in times of heightened psychological or physical stress.

Evaluation of Interventions. With regard to the particular significance of the very individual course of the disorder and response to therapy, e.g. Biederman et al. [13] suggest the following distinctions based on DSM-III-R: (1) syndromal remission: the patient no longer fulfils the criteria of the disorder (fewer than 8 of the 14 criteria), (2) symptomatic remission: the patient no longer fulfils the criteria of subcategorial disorder (fewer than 5 symptoms), and (3) functional remission: the patient has fewer than 5 symptoms and no longer exhibits impairments.

In DSM-IV, allowances are also made for differing courses, wherein it is advised that all patients who display symptoms at present, but do no longer fulfill all criteria, should be classified under the specification 'in partial remission'.

Comorbidity. Particularly in the case of adults, an associated problem is that a broad spectrum of comorbid disorders is possible [see Klein and Mannuzza, chapter 7]. Some of these disorders (e.g. depression) can develop secondarily as a result of years of frustration and failure experienced by the patient. The identification of comorbidity sometimes causes problems because other psychiatric disorders also have or can have their roots in adolescence or early adulthood. Relevant here are for example personality disorder, above all borderline personality disorder, antisocial personality disorder but also other psychiatric disorders such as obsessive-compulsive disorder or schizophrenia. These can be present as comorbid disorders, however they should also be thought of as differential diagnosis (see below).

Impairments. The associated impairments of the disorder can be more difficult to discern in adulthood. Activities, above all in the workplace, vary in the nature of their demands on attention, ability to plan, structuring and so on. Patients often find an 'ecological' niche, in which the symptoms do not have any or only a limited effect on their life [see Rösler, chapter 8]. The impairments resulting from ADHD symptoms often first become relevant and obvious when certain general frameworks change (e.g. change of workplace).

Rating Errors. As in the diagnosis of other psychiatric disorders, general diagnostic errors of judgment also have a bearing here (e.g. false conclusions, non-observance of criteria). A particular relevant error of judgment in view of ADHD diagnostics however is what is known as informant bias [14]. Because the disorder is relatively well known, patients often arrive to the assessment already informed, have certain expectations and this prior knowledge can certainly have an influence on self-evaluation.

A further general source of error can arise due to hasty conclusions based on a single source of information (e.g. only self-evaluation of the patients [see 15]).

Differential Considerations. Adults, in particular, can also suffer from somatic illnesses, which produce symptoms similar to ADHD, e.g. hypo- or hyperthyreosis, diabetes or certain heart problems [see 14]. It is imperative to rule these out as a first step. Some further important aspects are explicitly advised for consideration [see 14]:

- *ADHD, predominantly inattentive type*

It is necessary here to exclude the possibility that symptoms are a sign of another psychiatric disorder or somatic illness.

- *Substance abuse/dependence*

Frequent comorbidity with substance abuse makes it difficult to resolve the issue of whether the supposed ADHD symptoms are not due to substance abuse. An analysis of the chronology of the psychopathology helps here. ADHD appears, as a rule, before other psychiatric disorders, which usually only manifest themselves later.

- *Differential diagnosis from other psychiatric disorders*

It is necessary here, as already mentioned, to consider the variety of comorbid disorders as well as alternative diagnoses, above all anxiety disorders, depression, borderline personality disorder or bipolar affective disorders and particularly juvenile mania. Personality disorders are of special interest. ADHD in adulthood has a similar status to personality disorders:

- Because of the high comorbidity [see Klein and Mannuzza, chapter 7] they are often overlooked initially because other disorders are more prominent (e.g. depressive disorders).

Table 2. Multimodal assessment

Databases	Basic units of consideration (perspectives: e.g. biochemical, physiological, psychological, social, ecological)
Sources of data	Data provider (e.g. patient, therapist, nursing staff, reference person, neutral observer)
Functional ranges	Partial aspect within a database (e.g. psychological databases: experiences, behavior, feeling, working capacity)

- Both disorders show a range of common characteristics, such as e.g. early onset as well as impairments in different functional areas.
- It is particularly important to consider the substantial overlap at criteria level, above all to borderline personality disorder.

Multimodal Assessment and Diagnostic Process

With consideration to the particular aspects of ADHD diagnosis detailed in the previous section, a brief overview now follows of the diagnostic process, which has a multimodal diagnosis as its specific character. It is generally agreed that human behavior and experience have to be recorded in a multimodal way (other terms occasionally used: multimethod, multimethodically). Thus, distinctions are made between the following aspects [16]: databases, sources of data and functional ranges (table 2). One further aspect should be added: the type of instruments which are used to assess the relevant aspects of interest (e.g. rating scales, achievement tests). *Multimodal assessment* can be understood as a *general framework* which has to be specified for the concrete assessment of individual persons or groups of persons, making it necessary to select specific instruments [17]. The choice should be made according to specific criteria. On the one hand, methodological aspects should play a central role (e.g. high psychometric quality, especially reliability and validity). At the same time, conceptual considerations should be of equal relevance. This means that instruments should be used which allow the characterization of the important aspects of the construct in question.

A multimodal approach is generally required for evaluation of for example psychotherapy and psychotropic drug research in order to cope with the complexity of the phenomena studied. It is necessary to choose a multimodal approach in order to do justice to the complexity of this area and to account for the variance in the degree of exactness in databases and data providers as well as functional ranges. Furthermore, the necessity of a multimodal approach arises from the need to reduce investigator-dependent rating bias and results in the inclusion of different perspectives. With regard to the self-rating scales, bias may include acquiescence, central tendency or

Table 3. Multimodal assessment of ADHD in adults: psychological database and data sources

Psychological database	Data sources				
	patient	therapist	significant others	independent rater	other (e.g. case reports, school record, work references)
Current feelings	✓	(✓)	(✓)	(✓)	
Past feelings	✓	(✓)	(✓)	(✓)	
Current performance	✓	(✓)	✓	✓	
Past performance	✓	(✓)	✓	(✓)	✓
Current behavior	✓	✓	✓	✓	
Past behavior	✓	(✓)	✓	(✓)	✓

✓ = Evaluation possible; (✓) = evaluation only partly possible.

social desirability, on the level of observer-rating scales it may come from insufficient experience with the scale, response sets like generosity error or leniency error. In planning a study, care has to be taken that it contains sufficient distinctive measures to cover the domain of interest, but also that it does not include redundant measures (reduction of statistical power).

When these considerations are transferred to the field of ADHD, it can almost be argued that ADHD is prototypical for a multimodal diagnosis:

Database. On the biological or neurobiological data level there are, in the interim, a number of interesting results from the fields of neurophysiology or neuroimaging [see Baehne and Fallgatter, chapter 4, and Schneider et al., chapter 5]. As regards the psychological data level, problems can be seen in almost all areas such as experience, behavior and performance. On the social data level, (certain) conspicuous attributes are already detectable in the development of the person (e.g. outsider, few childhood friendships) which is equally noted as a consequence of the disorder (e.g. few friends). Additionally, the ecological data level, which is not sufficiently considered in most disorders, is of significance here. Individual problems such as financial problems, e.g. through job loss, should be mentioned [see Rösler, chapter 8].

Data Sources. Other than in hardly any other psychiatric disorder, all available data sources are important (table 3). Every data source can contribute specific information to the various aspects of the disorder from its particular perspective. The main data source is certainly the patient. Also of high significance is information from significant others. Ideally, information should be obtained from people who have current contact with the patient (e.g. partner, parents, close friends, siblings) as well as people who knew the patient well as a child (e.g. parents, uncle, aunt, older siblings). In some cases, however, this must be abandoned because such people are not available or the patient does not consent to others being questioned. As in other psychiatric disorders, the relation between self- and observer rating is of particular significance. Therefore, this relationship is briefly looked into in more detail. Following a variety of method studies, one can generally assume today that the two do not replace each other, but rather have a complementary function [17]. Achenbach et al. [18], in a meta-analysis of 108 studies, arrived at the result that even parallel instruments, that is instruments with the same content, only show moderate correlations (substance use $r_{mean} = 0.68$, internalizing problems $r_{mean} = 0.42$, externalizing problems $r_{mean} = 0.44$), non-parallel instruments correlated even less ($r_{mean} = 0.30$). Self- and observer rating allow specific aspects of each involved disorder to be represented from a different perspective.

With regard to the value of self- and observer rating in the context of ADHD, it is advisable to be aware of some particular aspects. An added complication in the field of ADHD is that in using both groups of instruments, not only the present symptomatology must be collected, but the symptomatology of the past must also be collected retrospectively. In clinical practice it is often shown, according to Murphy und Gordon [14], that also in ADHD different data sources do not correspond. Significant differences can arise between patient, parents and relatives in the evaluation of ADHD symptoms or in the perception of the severity of the associated impairments which result. Parents of adult ADHD patients, for example, often report fewer symptoms than the patient himself. There can be various reasons for this, such as simple forgetfulness about the pathology after time has elapsed. Other possible explanations can be that cultural factors, feelings of guilt or the presence of relatively less visible impairment in contrast to siblings are responsible for this.

Although self-evaluation constitutes a central function, its value and significance are currently controversially discussed in the literature. Some interesting methodical aspects are briefly mentioned here. Murphy and Schachar [19] compared self- and observer rating in two studies. They found high correlations in total (range 0.54–0.85) and thus concluded that patients can rate both their past and present ADHD symptoms in a relatively reliable manner. Rösler et al. [20] found similar results for an ADHD self-rating scale, which was compared to an ADHD expert rating (ADHD-DC). Both scales include the 18 diagnostic criteria from DSM-IV. The intraclass correlations on criteria level were between 0.41 and 0.92, for the area of attention deficit, hyperactivity and impulsivity between 0.75 and 0.84. The total score amounted to 0.87. Barkley et al. [9] concluded from the results of their methodical oriented study, however, that one should be rather cautious concerning retrospective self-reports [see also 15]. Glutting et al. [21] investigated the dimensionality of ADHD symptoms in self- and observer rating (patients and parents as data sources). It was shown that there is a three-dimensional solution (inattention, hyperactivity, impulsivity) in self-rating, however, only a two-dimensional solution (inattention, hyperactivity/impulsivity) in observer rating. This means that ADHD patients, in contrast to patients of other psychiatric disorders, seem better placed than their significant others to distinguish between different aspects of their disorder.

As well as results from self- and observer-rating methods, additional information can be drawn upon and namely such information which has a bearing on the development history of the patient, most importantly reports of any possible earlier medical and psychological assessments or school reports. According to Weiss and Murray [22], information which can be extracted from school documents is of particular significance. School reports are of most importance here. The actual school achievement grades are of much less significance here than written comments and remarks. Important are references to attention and concentration (e.g. daydreamer, cannot focus attention), level of activity (e.g. keeps standing up in class, cannot sit still) or impulsivity (e.g. is disruptive, interrupts others, cannot wait his turn).

Constructs/Functional Areas. As in other psychiatric disorders, various constructs or function areas must be considered. This is exemplified by the psychological data level; the most important at time of assessment. The general constructs feelings, behavior and achievement are found again in various facets of the disorder such as affect, impulsivity, a heightened reagibility, hyperactivity or attention.

Methods of Information Gathering. In the gathering of relevant information, rating scales on psychopathology are the main resource available – as well as diagnostic interviews and general and neuropsychological achievement tests. In the case of medical methods, neuroimaging is the main method to mention [see Schneider et al., chapter 5], although this has hitherto been mostly of significance in research and less so in practical diagnostic issues.

There are various suggestions to be found in the literature, as to how the mentioned aspects in the diagnostic process are to be integrated and considered [see e.g. 14, 22, 23]. With consideration of these thoughts and the previous report, the diagnostic process could look as represented in figure 1.

Weiss et al. [23] suggest the following steps in the practical diagnostic procedure, which do not, however, necessarily occur in the mentioned sequence: clinical interview, assessment of symptoms of ADHD and use of rating scales, assessment of other psychiatric disorders, assessment in childhood, further psychological assessments as well as assessment of impairments.

Step 1: Clinical Interview. The clinical interview has the function of documenting the patient and his life history as well as his current observable behavior. It serves as an assessment of the ADHD symptoms and other disorders as well as a rating of the current level of functioning.

Step 2: Assessment of ADHD Symptoms and Use of Rating Scales. Rating scales in the form of self- and observer-rating scales can serve to quantify current as well as past symptoms.

Step 3: Assessment of Other Psychiatric Disorders. Because of the high comorbidity of ADHD with other psychiatric disorders, it is of utmost importance to screen, at least broadly, for other psychiatric disorders and in case of suspicion to systematically assess e.g. by means of a structured interview (see table 7).

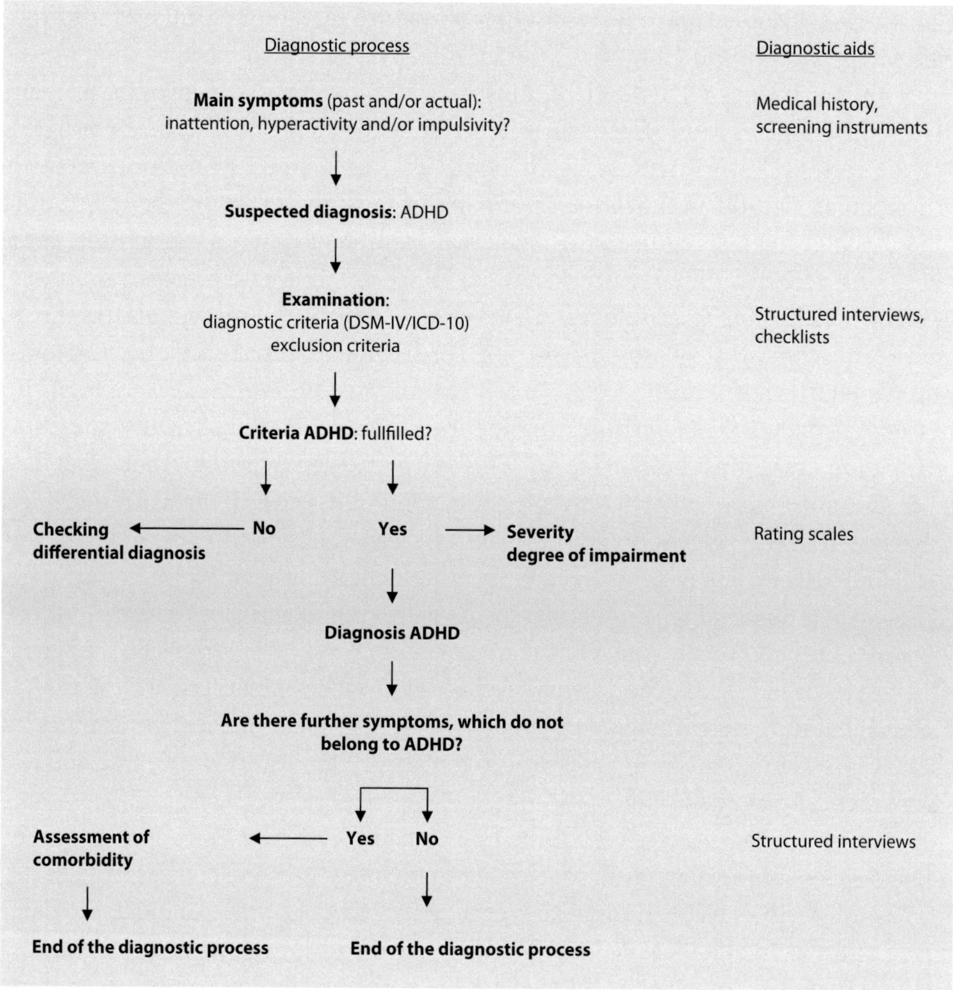

Fig. 1. Diagnostic process.

Step 4: Assessment of Symptoms in Childhood. The diagnosis of an ADHD in adulthood is based on the diagnostic findings of the history of the disorder in childhood. Adults with an ADHD often report very vibrant memories of childhood. Worth mentioning are for example emotional reactions from teachers and parents. If there are difficulties in remembering childhood, the investigator is dependent on additional sources of information. Reference to school reports sometimes generates valuable insights.

Step 5: Further Assessments. Although there are no definitive test procedures on the performance level for the diagnosis of an ADHD, they can provide supplementary information. To mention are for example psychological tests referring to achievement. These cannot, however, serve as a replacement for a clinical interview and the specific assessment and gathering of the psychopathology by means of specific scales.

Step 6: Assessment of Impairments. Because ADHD is attended by manifold impairments, the areas possibly affected such as quality of life, family situation or work, relationship, education as well as activities in everyday life should be differently assessed. Rating scales can be helpfully used here as well [see Rösler, chapter 8].

In summary, the diagnosis of an ADHD in adulthood is based on a clinical decision process; the diagnosis is ultimately a clinical diagnosis. This diagnosis is based on many facets which count for consideration in the context of the disorder, in which, above all, a comprehensive examination concerning psychopathology, functional impairments, extent of the disorder, onset of the illness and the absence of other illnesses are of utmost significance. All available data sources must be considered. It must be explicitly pointed out that up to now there are no neurobiological methods or diagnostic instruments (e.g. neuropsychological tests) which make a diagnosis of ADHD possible. We agree with Murphy and Adler [24, p. 12] that there is no litmus test (i.e. nor neuropsychological test or test battery, brain scan, or blood test) that can reliably diagnose ADHD.

Assessment Instruments

Overview

The following general assessment objectives are of significance in the ADHD context:

- Because of the high prevalence of the disorder, screening in different contexts has an important function. This is important because most patients have not been diagnosed in childhood and adolescence.
- For this reason, a retrospective diagnosis is usually necessary as well, that is to determine if a diagnosis in child and adolescence is possible using existing information.
- If the patient has been diagnosed earlier, it is necessary to verify the earlier diagnosis made or to test if the criteria are also currently fulfilled.
- If this is the case, the next step is to quantify the current degree of severity.
- Under treatment conditions, it is necessary to assess changes over the course of time, as well as the
- assessment of impairments at the start as well as over the course of the treatment and
- if applicable, the assessment of secondary symptoms as for example the degree of depression or anxiety.

Of central significance first of all is the question of to what extent an ADHD is actually present. Rating and assessment of an ADHD should therefore clarify these fundamental questions [14]: (1) Is there clear indication that the ADHD-typical symptoms

Table 4. Important aspects in diagnosing ADHD in adults

– General psychiatric history
– Medical examination
– Developmental, school, family and treatment history
– Assessment of past and actual ADHD symptomatology using standardized instruments
– Assessment of past and actual impairments in different areas of living
– Assessment of comorbid disorders
– If necessary neuropsychological assessment

For more information, see Weiss and Murray [22] and Murphy and Gordon [14].

had already emerged in childhood? (2) Is there clear indication that significant and consistent impairments in various areas have developed for the patient due to ADHD symptoms? (3) Are there other explanations for the ADHD which make the clinical picture more coherent? (4) For patients who fulfill the criteria for an ADHD, are there indications that other comorbid disorders are present?

The clinical interview is the core of the diagnostic process. It is a matter of making a detailed assessment of the various components of the past and current life situation (table 4). The following aspects at least should therein be covered: Assessment of symptomatology, development history and assessment of physical illness, school and work history, preexisting psychiatric disorders including prescribed medication, dosage and response, social adaptation, family history relating to ADHD or other psychiatric disorders, legal transgressions, the general level of functioning in everyday life. In the assessment of current and past history, there are a range of resources available, for example in the form of structured checklists for medical history. The best known is that from Barkley [25]. Among other factors, it includes the assessment of family history, school development and the family history of psychiatric illness. Although it was primarily designed for children and adolescents, it can also be used to great advantage in the adult domain.

In response to the mentioned questions, the examiner has nowadays a range of diagnostic methods available as resources although ADHD in adults is a 'young' disorder in comparison to other psychiatric disorders. When one attempts to systematize the methods, the following distinction can be made: (1) self-rating scales, (2) observer-rating scales and (3) diagnostic interviews for classification.

The following tables include examples of just a few of the multitude of methods which are now available [see also 14, 23, 25, 26]. Only those instruments were selected for which sufficient data is available to confirm their reliability and validity.

Self-Rating Scales

Under the term *self-rating scales* one understands methods in which the entire process of rating of the (involved) phenomena is carried out by the patient. Self-rating

Table 5. Self-rating scales for adults (examples)

Instrument (abbr., authors)	Characteristics	Different languages	Time to complete min	Interpretation
Adult ADHD Self-Report Scale v1.1 (ASRS v1.1; WHO) or ASRS V1.1. Screener (Adler et al.; WHO)	18 items of DSM-IV	Yes	5–10	+
ADHD Self-Rating (ADHS-SB; Rösler et al.)	18 items according to DSM-IV and ICD-10, 4 additional items (e.g. disability)	No	5–10	+
Wender Utah Rating Scale (WURS; Wender; Retz-Junginger et al.)	61 or 25 items, Utah criteria	Yes	10–12	+
Conners' Adult ADHD Rating Scale Self-Report (CAARS-SR; Conners)	Self-rating scale, different versions, among other things DSM-IV criteria	No	10–20	+
Brown Attention-Deficit Disorder Scales (Brown ADD Scales)	Self-rating scale, 5 dimensions	No	15–30	+

+ = Norms or cut-off-scores available. For further information, see Rösler et al. [26].

methods have the advantage that they, among other points, are time-economical in use and allow assessment of multifaceted areas. Disadvantages to mention are, among others, the susceptibility to errors of rating bias or the limitations of the application (e.g. only to a certain severity level of the disorder).

Among self-rating scales, a distinction should be made between those in which the retrospective assessment of ADHD symptoms is concerned and those dealing with current symptoms. In table 5, examples of self-rating scales in the context of an ADHS diagnosis are found. When a concrete suspicion does not yet exist or patients do not come at their own initiative with a request for an assessment, the use of so-called screening instruments is appropriate. These serve as a way of 'filtering out' risk persons, who can then be more closely examined. In the next phase of the diagnostic process, further self-rating scales can then be used with the objective of gathering information for the rating of diagnostic criteria or assessing the severity of the current symptomatology.

Observer-Rating Scales

Observer-rating scales are based on patient statements and observations from a trained rater. The rating of the existence of symptoms for example is however made entirely by the rater. In studies, as a rule, observer-rating methods are chosen as the main outcome criterion because they, among other points, allow a differentiated

Table 6. Observer-rating scales (incl. interviews) for adults (examples)

Instrument (abbr., authors)	Characteristics	Different languages	Time to complete min	Interpretation
Wender-Reimher Interview (WRI; Wender; Rösler et al.)	Interview, 7 dimensions according to Wender and Reimher	Yes	30	+
Conners' Adult ADHD Rating Scale Observer Report (CAARS-OR; Conners)	Observer-rating scale, different versions, among other things DSM criteria	Yes	10–20	+
Brown ADD Rating Scale (Brown ADD-RS)	Observer-rating scale, 40 items, 5 dimensions	Yes	15	+

+ = Norms or cut-off scores available. For more information, see Rösler et al. [26].

picture of psychopathology, are more sensitive to measure change and are also able to be used in severe cases of the disorder. Established observer-rating scales in the context of ADHD diagnostics are found in table 6. These can also be distinguished by the degree to which they allow retrospective assessment or allow the assessment of the current disorder and its severity. In order to reduce the major sources of error in the diagnostic process, observation and information variance, the use of interviews for information gathering has proven to be of value. Through the allocation of questions drawn from individual diagnostic criteria or symptoms, the information variance is reduced, and through assignment of rating of the collected information, the observation variance is reduced.

Diagnostic Interviews

Observer-rating scales and therein associated interviews must be distinguished from interviews used for classificatory diagnosis. These have the objective either to diagnose an ADHD or a comorbid disorder. Interviews for diagnosis of an ADHD are rare. The best known is Conners' Adult ADHD Diagnostic Interview for DSM-IV (CAADID [27]). The interview consists of two parts: In part I, information related to four areas is collected: demographic history, developmental course, ADHD risk factors, comorbidity screening questions. Part II of the CAADID examines if the patient meets the DSM-IV criteria of ADHD (in childhood and currently).

Comorbidity in ADHD seems to be, on the evidence of previous epidemiological studies, the rule rather than the exception [see Klein and Mannuzza, chapter 7]. In the assessment of comorbidity, a range of structured and standardized interviews have proved of value; they are also included in table 7. These are instruments which also find application in the context of psychiatric assessment.

Table 7. Diagnostic interviews for ADHD and comorbid disorders (examples)

Instrument (abbr., authors)	Characteristics	Time to complete min	Different languages	Classification system
ADHD-specific				
Wender-Reimher Interview (WRI; Wender; Rösler et al.)	Structured interview	30	Yes	No
Conners' Adult ADHD Diagnostic Interview for DSM-IV (CAADID; Epstein et al.)	Structured interview	90	No	DSM-IV
General				
Structured Clinical Interview for DSM-IV (SKID-I and –II; First et al.)	Structured interview	60–90	Yes	DSM-IV
Schedules for Clinical Assessment in Neuropsychiatry (SCAN; WHO)	Structured interview	90–120	Yes	ICD-10
Mini International Neuropsychiatric Interview (MINI; Sheehan et al.)	Structured interview	15–20	Yes	ICD-10/ DSM-IV
Composite International Diagnostic Interview (CIDI; WHO)	Standardized interview	60–90	Yes	ICD-10/ DSM-IV

For more information, see Rösler et al. [26] and Sajatovic and Ramirez [36].

Other Important Domains

As well as ADHD symptoms in the narrow sense and possible comorbid disorder(s), further domains are to be considered as listed in table 8. Proven helpful to the extensive description of the problematic have been general psychopathological rating scales as for example the SCL-90-R as multidimensional instrument or syndrome-specific procedures of assessment (e.g. the severity of depression). Because ADHD is accompanied by multifaceted impairments in various areas of life, these should be sufficiently broad and differentially assessed. This is true on one hand for the impact on quality of life (for the specific assessment of quality of life in ADHD, see Brod et al. [28]) particularly, however, for the assessment of constraints in various aspects of life (work partnership/relationship, families, etc.). Also habitual aspects of personality should be considered in the context of an ADHD (e.g. impulsiveness, disproportionate risk-taking).

A psychological assessment (general or neuropsychological performance assessment) can form a significant proportion of the clinical assessment. Previous

Table 8. Relevant areas in the assessment of ADHD in adults: instruments (examples)

Area	Instrument (abbr., author)	Characteristics
General psychopathology	Symptom Checklist (SCL-90-R; Derogatis)	Self-rating 90 items 9 dimensions 3 global scores
	Beck Depression Inventory (BDI, Beck et al.)	Self-rating 21 items Total score depression
	Montgomery-Åsberg Depression Rating Scale (MADRS; Montgomery & Åsberg)	Observer rating 10 items Total score depression
	Beck Anxiety Inventory (BAI; Beck et al.)	Self-rating 21 items Total score anxiety
General mental health status	Clinical Global Impressions (CGI; Guy)	Observer rating Global score of illness (severity) Global score improvement
Disability	Sheehan Disability Scale (SDS; Sheehan)	Self-rating 3 items (social life, work, family)
Relationship	Dyadic Adjustment Scale (DAS; Spanier)	Self-rating 32 items 4 dimensions
Personality	Eysenck Impulsiveness Questionnaire (I7; Eysenck et al.)	Self-rating 54 items 3 dimensions (impulsivity, venturesomeness, empathy)
Social adaptation	Social and Occupational Functioning Assessment Scale (SOFAS; APA)	Observer rating Global score DSM-IV (optional)
Quality of life	World Health Organisation Quality of Life Assessment Instrument (WHO-QOL-100; WHO)	Self-rating 100 items 6 subscales
	SF-36 Health Survey (SF-36; Ware)	Self- and observer rating 36 Items 8 subscales

For further information, see APA [35] and Sajatovic and Ramirez [36].

studies have shown that no single test or battery of tests has had a predictive validity or specificity regarding reliable assessment of an ADHD. Neuropsychological examinations alone can never provide the basis for an ADHD diagnosis, but they do provide in some individual cases, however, indications of the extent of impairments such as sustained attention, working memory or executive functioning. Established methods of neuropsychological diagnostics can find application here [see 29, 30].

Although several methods now exist, the psychometric status of individual instruments is, however, often unclear. One must then demand that the instruments are sufficiently evaluated. Several guidelines exist [e.g. 31] that can be used by practitioners and scientists to select instruments that are suitable for their purposes. The guidelines can also be used to evaluate the appropriateness of an instrument that is in use or proposed for use.

Prevalence

In the epidemiology of ADHD in adulthood, only rather approximate estimates exist so far (see above). There are various reasons for this. Among others, the following points should be mentioned: (1) ADHD in adulthood has only been a focus of interest in research for a few years; (2) no explicit, official operationalization of the disorder for adulthood exists (neither ICD-10 nor DSM-IV), and (3) the disorder is therefore not included in interviews used in epidemiological studies.

A number of prospective studies have followed children with ADHD into late adolescence or early adulthood in order to estimate the prevalence of persistence [4]. Controversy has surrounded the resulting persistence estimates because they depend on the criteria used to select the sample, the edition of DSM used to make the diagnosis of adults, and whether adult symptom assessment was based on self-reports or informant reports [4]. A relatively large number of studies have been published that estimate the persistence of ADHD throughout adolescence and adulthood [5] and the rate of ADHD varies from one study to the next. Mick et al. [5] summarize the studies depending on the different versions of DSM: (1) DSM-II diagnosis at baseline: range persistence 4–86%, (2) DSM-III diagnosis at baseline: range persistence 34–80%, and (3) DSM-III-R diagnosis at baseline: range persistence 58–85%.

Using this data, they computed combined estimate rates for the three diagnostic systems: 40% for DSM-II, 52% for DSM-III, and 74% for DSM-III-R.

In contrast to many studies of the prevalence of ADHD in children, estimates of the prevalence of adult ADHD have been indirect and rely on three types of studies [6]: (1) longitudinal follow-up studies of ADHD children into adulthood; (2) community surveys using samples of convenience, and (3) family studies of childhood ADHD that examined the prevalence of ADHD in the adult relatives of non-ADHD comparison children.

Table 9. Prevalence of ADHD in adults

Authors	Method and sample; diagnostic system	Results
Faraone and Biederman [6]	Telephone survey of 966 randomly selected adults; DSM-IV Interviewer: persons experienced in the administration of telephone surveys	Narrow screening diagnosis – Combined subtype: 1.1% – Inattentive subtype: 0.7% – Hyperactive-impulsive subtype: 1.1% Broad screening diagnosis – Combined subtype: 6.9% – Inattentive subtype: 5.8% – Hyperactive-impulsive subtype: 3.7%
Kessler et al. [7]	Screen for adult ADHD in a probability subsample (n = 3,199) of 18- to 44-year-old respondents in the National Comorbidity Survey, follow-up interview with 154 respondents; DSM-IV Interviewer: professional survey staff	Estimated prevalence 4.4%

Attempts to estimate prevalence by extrapolating from childhood prevalence estimates linked with adult persistence estimates or by directly estimating prevalence in small samples of adults or college students have yielded prevalence estimates in the range of 1–6% [4, 7].

Assuming an example prevalence rate of 5–10% in children [8] and the assumption of a persistence from 50 to 60% in adulthood [e.g. 9], an estimate of prevalence amounts to around 2–4% in adulthood. Evidence from newer studies suggests that these estimates are probably rather too low (table 9). Faraone and Biederman [6] completed a telephone survey of 966 randomly selected adults. They estimate a prevalence rate of 2.9% for so-called narrow ADHD and 16.4% for broad ADHD. Kessler et al. [7] found in their National Comorbidity Survey Replication an estimated prevalence of 4.4% (total sample n = 3,199, age 18–44). In summary, the data from previous and current studies suggests that ADHD is a common psychiatric disorder.

Summary and Perspectives

There is, in the meantime, clear support to show that ADHD is not an 'artificial' category, but a valid diagnostic entity, which experienced clinicians can reliably assess. A comprehensive and thorough examination is essential, which, above all, considers critical aspects of the past, the current level of functioning, the extent of impairments and possible alternative explanations.

Although diagnostics of adult ADHD has a young history, several diagnostic instruments now exist which serve as important building blocks for a reliable ADHD diagnosis. Because the ADHD diagnosis is ultimately a clinical diagnosis, assessment instruments fulfill an important function in addition to medical history. This is also true of scales to determine severity of current symptoms. No single instrument can provide a diagnosis!

Although there are already many instruments available, there are currently still many deficits which should be mentioned:

- There are no official, generally accepted guidelines regarding the evaluation of diagnostic instruments in the domain of ADHD for adults.
- There is as yet no gold standard, but rather a range of competing instruments which often makes the comparison of study results difficult. With reference to the comparability and generalizability of study results for case studies as well as therapy studies, a standardized assessment battery would be desirable, in which, above all, a standardization regarding the main outcomes should be strived for.
- Method studies (e.g. multitrait-multimethod analysis, MTMM [32]) should provide information about which instrument(s) should be used in future.
- On the level of scales which determine severity, no instrument has as yet, proven sufficiently sensitive to measure change.
- Other than a few exceptions [e.g. 33, 34], almost no norms for representative samples of healthy individuals and clinical samples exist.

In addition, general problems of diagnostics of ADHD still exist, independently of individual instruments. The following are particularly worth mentioning:

- The need for adaptation of diagnostic criteria for adulthood in the revision of the current classification systems ICD-10 und DSM-IV is of central significance. As the introduction of ICD-11 und DSM-V is set for approximately 2012, there still remains sufficient time for this step.
- Diagnostic criteria should be included in diagnostic interviews such as e.g. SCID or CIDI (table 7), either as an add-on module or as an obligatory module.
- As also in the case of many other disorders (e.g. personality disorders) the question of the additional dimensional description to categorical perspective should be discussed. This can be executed in various ways (e.g. number of criteria fulfilled or by means of a rating scale [see also 11]).

Clinical assessment of ADHD requires more than merely deciding whether the disorder is present or not. Since treatment decisions and evaluation are usually not only based on diagnoses, the demand arises for a multimodal assessment of the individual patient in practice as well as research. In general, different sources of data, databases and functional ranges are to be taken into consideration in describing the patients [17]. This is one of the main important aspects in diagnosing ADHD in adults and the basis for reliable epidemiological data and in clinical routine for an appropriate therapy.

References

1 American Psychiatric Association: Diagnostic and Statistical Manual of Mental Disorders, ed 4. Washington, APA, 1994.

2 World Health Organization: The ICD-10 Classification of Mental and Behavioural Disorders: Diagnostic Criteria for Research. Geneva, WHO, 1994.

3 Faraone SV, Spencer T, Aleardi M, Pagano C, Biederman J: Meta-analysis of the efficacy of methylphenidate for treating attention-deficit/hyperactivity disorder. J Clin Psychopharmacol 2004;24:24–29.

4 Kessler RC, Adler LA, Barkley R, Biederman J, Conners CK, Faraone SV, Greenhill LL, Jaeger S, Secnik K, Spencer T, Uestün TB, Zaslavsky AM: Patterns and predictors of attention-deficit/hyperactivity disorder persistence into adulthood: results from the National Comorbidity Survey Replication. Biol Psychiatry 2005;57:1441–1451.

5 Mick E, Faraone SV, Biederman J, Spencer TJ: The course and outcome of attention-deficit/hyperactivity disorder. Primary Psychiatry 2004;11:42–48.

6 Faraone SV, Biederman J: What is the prevalence of adult ADHD? Results of a population screen of 966 adults. J Atten Disord 2005;9:384–391.

7 Kessler RC, Adler L, Ames M, Barkley RA, Birnbaum H, Greenberg P, Johnston JA, Spencer T, Uestün TB: The prevalence and effects of adult attention-deficit/hyperactivity disorder on work performance in a normally representative sample of workers. JOEM 2006;47:565–572.

8 Faraone SV, Sergeant J, Gillberg C, Biederman J: The worldwide prevalence of ADHD: Is it an American condition? World Psychiatry 2003;2:104–113.

9 Barkley RA, Fischer M, Smallish L, Fletcher K: The persistence of attention-deficit/hyperactivity disorder into young adulthood as a function of reporting source and definition disorder. J Abnorm Psychol 2002;111:279–289.

10 Faraone SV, Biederman J, Spencer T, Mick E, Kurray K, Petty C, Adamson JJ, Motuteaux MC: Diagnosing adult attention deficit hyperactivity disorder: Are late onset and subthreshold diagnoses valid? Am J Psychiatry 2006;163:1720–1729.

11 Helzer JE, Kraemer HC, Krueger RF: The feasibility and need for dimensional psychiatric diagnosis. Psychol Med 2006;36:1671–1680.

12 Faraone SV, Biederman J, Feighner JA, Monuteaux MC: Assessing symptoms of attention deficit hyperactivity disorder in children and adults: Which is more valid? J Consult Clin Psychol 2000;68:830–842.

13 Biederman JJ, Mick E, Faraone SV: Age-dependent decline of symptoms of attention deficit hyperactivity disorder: impact of remission definition and subtype. Am J Psychiatry 2000;157:816–818.

14 Murphy KR, Gordon M: Assessment of adults with ADHD; in Barkley RA (ed): Attention-Deficit Hyperactivity Disorder. New York, Guilford Press, 2006, pp 425–450.

15 McCann BS, Roy-Byrne P: Screening and diagnostic utility of self-report attention deficit disorder scales in adults. Compr Psychiatry 2004;45:175–183.

16 Baumann U, Eckmann F, Stieglitz RD: Self-rating data as a selecting factor in clinical trials of psychotropic drug. Eur Arch Psychiatry Neurol Sci 1985;235:65–70.

17 Stieglitz RD: Multimodal assessment (including triangulation); in Fernandez-Ballesteros R (ed): Encyclopedia of Psychological Assessment. London, Sage, 2003, pp 606–610.

18 Achenbach TM, Krukowski RA, Dumenci L, Ivanova MY: Assessment of adult psychopathology: meta-analyses and implications of cross-informant correlations. Psychol Bull 2005;131:361–382.

19 Murphy P, Schachar R: Use of self-ratings in the assessment of symptoms of attention-deficit hyperactivity disorder in adults. Am J Psychiatry 2000;157:1156–1159.

20 Rösler M, Retz W, Retz-Junginger P, Thome J, Supprian T, Nissen T, Stieglitz RD, Blocher D, Hengesch G, Trott GE: Instrumente zur Diagnostik der Aufmerksamkeitsdefizit-/Hyperaktivitätsstörung im Erwachsenenalter: Selbstbeurteilungsskala (ADHS-SB) und Diagnose Checkliste (ADHS-CL). Nervenarzt 2004;75:888–895.

21 Glutting JJ, Youngstrom EA, Watkins MW: ADHD and college students: exploratory and confirmatory factor structures with student and parent data. Psychol Assess 2005;17:44–55.

22 Weiss M, Murray C: Assessment and management of attention-deficit hyperactivity disorder in adults. CMAJ 2003;186:715–722.

23 Weiss M, Trokenberg Hechtman L, Weiss G: ADHD in Adulthood: a Guide to Current Theory, Diagnosis, and Treatment. Baltimore, John Hopkins University, 1999.

24 Murphy KR, Adler LA: Assessing attention-deficit/hyperactivity disorder in adults: Focus on rating scales. J Clin Psychiatry 2004;65(suppl 3):12–17.

25 Barkley RA: Attention-Deficit Hyperactivity Disorder. A Handbook for Diagnosis and Treatment, ed 2. New York, Guilford Press, 1998.

26 Rösler M, Retz W, Thome J, Schneider M, Stieglitz RD, Falkai P: Psychopathological rating scales for the diagnostic use in adult attention-deficit/hyperactivity disorder. Eur Arch Psychiatry Clin Neurosci 2006;256(suppl 1):I/3-I/11.
27 Epstein J, Johnson DE, Conners CK: Conners' Adult ADHD Diagnostic Interview for DSM-IV (CAADID). New York, Multi-Health Systems, 2001.
28 Brod M, Perwien A, Adler L, Spencer T, Johnston J: Conceptualization and assessment of quality of life for adults with attention-deficit/hyperactivity disorder. Primary Psychiatry 2005;12:58–64.
29 Hervey AS, Epstein JN, Curry JF: Neuropsychology of adults with attention-deficit/hyperactivity disorder: a meta-analytic review. Neuropsychology 2004; 18:485–503.
30 Schoechlin C, Engel RR: Neuropsychological performance in adult attention-deficit hyperactivity disorder: meta-analysis of empirical data. Arch Clin Neuropsychol 2005;20:727–744.
31 Newman FL, Carpenter D: Guidelines for selecting psychological instruments for treatment outcome assessment; in Clarkin JF, Docherty JP (eds): Psychological and Biological Assessment at the Turn of the Century. Washington, APA, 1997, pp 59–78.
32 Saris W, Münnich A (eds): The multitrait-multimethod approach to evaluate measurement instruments. Budapest, Eötvös University Press, 1995.
33 Brown TE: Brown attention deficit scales. San Antonio, The Psychological Corporation, 2001.
34 Conners CK, Ehrhard D, Sparrow D: Conners' Adult ADHD Rating Scales (CAARS). New York, Multi-Health Systems, 1999.
35 American Psychiatric Association: Handbook of Psychiatric Measures. Washington, APA, 2000.
36 Sajatovic M, Ramirez LF: Rating scales in mental health, ed 2. Hudson, LexiComp, 2003.

Prof. Dr. rer. nat. Dipl.-Psych. Rolf-Dieter Stieglitz
Psychiatric Outpatient Department, University Hospital Basel
Petersgraben 4
CH–4031 Basel (Switzerland)
Tel. +41 61 265 5106, Fax +41 61 265 4588, E-Mail rstieglitz@uhbs.ch

Retz W, Klein RG (eds): Attention-Deficit Hyperactivity Disorder (ADHD) in Adults.
Key Issues in Mental Health. Basel, Karger, 2010, vol 176, pp 126–143

Comorbidity in Adult Attention-Deficit Hyperactivity Disorder

Rachel G. Klein · Salvatore Mannuzza

New York University Child Study Center, Department of Child and Adolescent Psychiatry, New York, N.Y., USA

Abstract

In cross-sectional studies, attention-deficit hyperactivity disorder (ADHD) in adults has been linked to the presence of several other psychiatric disorders. This diagnostic comorbidity is consistently found for antisocial personality disorder and also substance use disorders. There is great divergence in reports of comorbid anxiety and mood disorders. Quality of designs varies widely, limiting interpretation of conflicting results. Evidence suggests that men and women with ADHD present with similar patterns of comorbidity, regardless of whether they are referred or non-referred individuals. Prospective follow-up studies of children with ADHD into adulthood have generated similar findings of comorbidity: elevated rates of antisocial personality and substance use disorders, and divergent findings with regard to comorbidity of anxiety and mood disorders. There is very limited information about differences in comorbidity between children whose ADHD persists into adulthood and those in whom it remits (prognostic comorbidity). The sparse evidence from prospective longitudinal studies suggests that antisocial personality is predicted by the retention of ADHD into adulthood. Except for nicotine dependence, no other condition has emerged as a significant correlate of persistent ADHD.

In its broadest concept, comorbidity has been defined as 'any distinct additional clinical entity that has existed or that may occur during the clinical course of a patient who has the index disease under study' [1]. This definition includes disorders that are antecedent to, and those that are concurrent with, a specific condition. This broad definition has been refined further by Kaplan and Feinstein [2] in their discussion of comorbidity in internal medicine. They describe prognostic comorbidity as the risk conferred by one disease for another disease. In the population, the relationship between the index and 'comorbid' condition is not a random phenomenon. However, in referring to an individual, the term comorbidity is also used to denote the co-occurrence of disorders, whether or not their joint presence exceeds chance expectation in the population. In general medicine, comorbidity refers to the presence of conditions that represent discrete diseases. Even if they are causally related, the two diseases have distinct pathophysiology, and often require different interventions (as in the example of diabetes and renal disease). The concept of comorbidity has been important in medicine since it has major implications for understanding mechanisms of pathophysiology, for clinical care, and for prevention. However, ambiguities emerge when applying this framework to psychiatric disorders. As noted by Fyer et al. [3], internal medicine provides many instances of different pathologies leading to similar clinical syndromes, e.g. diabetes, but the identification of distinct pathologies enables their differentiation. In contrast, psychiatric disorders are defined by their clinical presentation. Problematically, psychiatric disorders are polythetic. They not only share diagnostic features, but almost never possess uniquely pathognomonic symptoms. In the absence of pathophysiological data, symptomatic definitions lead to a situation in which similar syndromal presentations have diverse underlying pathology. The heterogeneity inherent in psychiatric disorders may lead to findings of comorbidity that do not apply across the entire clinical population, and may result in 'pseudocomorbidity' [4]. Unfortunately, there are no means of identifying phenocopies (syndromes that look alike but have distinct etiologies, be they genetic, environmental, or otherwise influenced). This diagnostic imprecision likely leads to misleading inferences about comorbidity.

Comorbidity in psychiatry is highly prevalent, and has received a great deal of attention, due to its importance for clinical management and research. Knowledge that disorders often co-occur, either concurrently or sequentially, will shape diagnostic and therapeutic practice. For example, if we know that individuals with substance use disorders (SUDs) are relatively more likely to have or have had attention-deficit/hyperactivity disorder (ADHD), inquiry for ADHD will become routine in the assessment of patients with substance disorders, and treatment plans will consider addressing both conditions. As an example, a population study found that adults with ADHD had high rates of comorbid disorders (described below) and that, among the treated individuals, treatment had mostly been for another disorder rather than ADHD.

Research-wise, knowledge of comorbidity justifies efforts to identify common risk factors, causes, and fosters improved diagnostic classification by making distinctions within a disorder when it is comorbid and when it is not. For example, if SUD that is comorbid with ADHD differs from non-comorbid SUD with regard to risk factors, prognosis, treatment response, brain function, the nomenclature might be altered to reflect such distinctions. However, in order for reports of comorbidity to generate meaningful and fruitful findings, its magnitude must exceed chance co-occurrence. If it does not, much effort will be wasted in the investigation of its significance.

Diagnostic and Methodological Issues

The influence of symptomatic overlap across disorders has been discussed by many as a potential confounder in the study of psychiatric comorbidity in general, but it may be especially salient in ADHD. The cardinal symptoms of ADHD, restlessness, inattention and impulsivity, are highly non-specific, and occur in numerous conditions, even if they are not they are not defining clinical criteria. As a result, disorders may be comorbid due to lack of symptomatic specificity across various diagnoses. With regard to ADHD, problems of symptomatic overlap appear likely for depression and bipolar disorder since they explicitly include similar features, such as poor concentration, restlessness and, in the case of bipolar disorder, impulsivity. That symptom overlap is a significant issue is illustrated by a study by Millberger et al. [5], in which 53% of children with comorbid ADHD and bipolar disorder ceased to meet criteria for bipolar disorder when symptoms common to mania and ADHD were removed. Another diagnostic limitation is that, in the DSM [6], diverse symptomatic expressions of a dysfunction are encompassed by a single label. A case in point might be poor concentration. It is probable that the symptom has different clinical features when it occurs in the context of ADHD versus depression, but no information is given on this point, and clinicians are not alerted to distinguish among various forms of inattention. The same applies to other symptoms. This lack of clinical refinement is likely to influence estimates of comorbidity.

Another related methodological issue is the use of non-clinicians to determine psychiatric diagnoses. Individuals without clinical experience and training cannot make symptomatic distinctions, especially since clinical decisions rely on verbal questionnaires. This approach to diagnosis is also likely to inflate comorbidity since the presence of symptoms depends exclusively on the positive endorsement of fixed questions that may be interpreted differently by various people. This dilemma is illustrated by findings of very high rates of anxiety disorders in children with ADHD diagnosed via a structured interview by non-clinicians [7].

In sum, the nature of classification in psychiatry poses major dilemmas in establishing whether disorders represent distinct conditions, thereby complicating true identification of comorbidity. In addition, diagnostic approaches commonly utilized, such as the reliance on lay interviewers, likely lead to overestimates of comorbidity. At the same time, the potential contribution of comorbidity to our understanding of psychopathology is so diverse and potentially informative that it remains a major interest.

In this review, whose focus is on adult ADHD, we report on the broad concept of diagnostic comorbidity, i.e., the co-occurrence of adult ADHD with other diagnoses, and on prognostic comorbidity of childhood ADHD to adult psychopathology.

Study Designs and Estimates of Comorbidity

Besides diagnostic issues, differences in study designs also influence and possibly confound estimates of comorbidity. A number of studies have conducted cross-sectional evaluations of self-referred adults, often in adult ADHD clinics, to estimate prevalence of comorbid disorders. Others have assessed ADHD in adults with other psychiatric disorders (alcoholism, cocaine abuse, major depressive disorder, etc.). In these instances, the establishment of childhood ADHD relies on retrospective recall. It is generally acknowledged that children with ADHD are very poor observers and reporters of their difficulties, and that the diagnosis must rely on informants, typically parents and teachers. Can we expect children with ADHD to become accurate about early history some 20 years later? It is possible that, with age, people develop more objective appreciation of their childhood ADHD symptoms than they had at the time. In a systematic prospective study of recall of childhood ADHD, we found that 78% of 176 adults with confirmed ADHD in childhood, reported childhood symptoms of inattention, hyperactivity and/or impulsivity that qualified for a diagnosis of ADHD in childhood (most had been treated for extended periods, which should have enhanced correct recollection); in turn, 11% of 168 normal comparisons erroneously recalled childhood ADHD [8]. These findings of 0.78 sensitivity and 0.89 specificity appear encouraging. However, sensitivity varies as a function of base rate [9], consequently, the 0.78 sensitivity does not reflect the accuracy to be expected when the base rate of ADHD is low, as is the case in the general population. By applying a sensitivity rate of 0.78 to an adult population in which 5% truly had childhood ADHD, only 27% of those who report childhood ADHD will be accurately identified (positive predictive value). However, 99% of those judged not to have had ADHD would be correctly classified (negative predictive value) [8]. Thus, in a situation where ADHD is infrequent, the great majority of individuals who indicate that they had ADHD in childhood will be wrong. In contrast, accuracy will be much better in cases who do not indicate childhood ADHD.

Because of inherent limitations in retrospective recall, prospective longitudinal studies of children with established ADHD are much preferable. However, prospective studies also pose their own methodological problems. It is virtually impossible for longitudinal studies to gather information from all individuals in the entire original groups. Therefore, selective attrition becomes a major concern since the partial sample successfully followed may differ from the original cohort in ways that affect estimates of comorbidity. Some have found that missing cases had better outcomes [10], others have reported the opposite [11] and yet others find significant differences in childhood between retrieved and missing ADHD subjects [12].

Also limiting features of longitudinal studies may be the failure to have collected informative predictors in childhood, and changes in the diagnostic definition of ADHD over time. These complicate the relevance of prospective studies that span several decades. At the same time, provided that the early information was systematically obtained and comprehensive (e.g., multiple informants and ratings, psychiatric evaluations, etc.), the onset of the disorder in childhood is assured. Another hindrance to meaningful long-term studies is the need for appropriate controls identified at the time the ADHD children were identified. The full complement of optimal design features is scarce in longitudinal studies of children with ADHD into adulthood.

Concurrent Comorbidity

The current nomenclature includes three types of ADHD, combined, predominantly inattentive, and predominantly hyperactive-impulsive types. This convention enhances further the heterogeneity and polythetic nature of ADHD. Our goal is to address comorbidity in ADHD, combined type. Most major studies have restricted their sample to this ADHD type. An exception is the Boston group that reports on the course of combined and predominantly inattentive types, without distinction.

The evidence on comorbidity in adult ADHD stems from cross-sectional clinical studies, and prospective studies that have followed children with ADHD into adulthood. As shown in table 1, these differ in multiple ways such as retrieval rate, blindness, etc. [10, 12–17]. Despite these differences, certain findings regarding mental status have been consistent. For one, all longitudinal studies have found that ADHD persisted into adulthood in a significant proportion of ADHD children. However, the magnitude of estimates of that proportion has varied widely (7% of probands reporting the full or partial syndrome at follow-up in the New York Study [16, 17] to 58% in the Boston study [12]). Possible reasons for these discrepancies are discussed elsewhere [18]. In addition, all prospective studies have shown that children with ADHD, compared to children without the disorder, have elevated rates of antisocial personality disorder (APD) in adulthood [10, 12–17], and three of the five studies report increased risk for SUD (described below) (table 1). Findings for other conditions are inconsistent. In each section, we present clinical reports of adults with ADHD first, followed by prospective longitudinal studies of children/adolescents with ADHD into adulthood.

Antisocial Personality Disorder

As shown in table 2, Downey et al. [19] and Torgersen et al. [20] have reported rates of 13 and 44% of APD in adults with ADHD, respectively. Since these investigations did not include a comparison group of non-ADHD adults, the specific relationship between ADHD and APD is obscure. The great dissimilarity in prevalence of APD between the two studies raises questions about methodological differences in establishing diagnoses, including the equivalence of the ADHD samples. Schubiner et al. [21], who evaluated randomly selected adult inpatients from two substance abuse treatment facilities, found that those with ADHD, compared to those without ADHD, had significantly higher rates of APD (69 vs. 29%, $p < 0.001$). This finding suggests that, among substance abusers, APD is also related to adult ADHD. In contrast, Murphy et al. [22] failed to find elevated rates of APD among adults attending ADHD clinics relative to adults without ADHD in the community (4 and 0%, respectively). In our prospective study of boys with ADHD (ages 6–12; mean age 8 years) followed into adulthood (mean age 25 years), 17 of 176 (10%) retained ADHD to at least age 18. As indicated in table 1, rates of APD among the 17 adults with ADHD were strikingly more prevalent than among the 168 non-ADHD comparisons (47 vs. 3%, $p < 0.001$) [23].

Table 1. Prospective, controlled studies of the course and outcome of children with ADHD followed into adulthood

Principal investigators	Location of study	Initial sample	n at FU	% childhood	Age at FU	FU interviewer		Person interviewed	Major outcome findings of adult mental status (ADHD refers to ongoing, at FU)
						clinician	blind		
Barkley and Fischer[a]	Milwaukee (USA)	Clinic	147	93	21	No	No	Parent Subject	1) P>C- ADHD, APD, MDD, PAPD, HPD, BPD 2) P=C- Alc, SUD, AD
Biederman[b]	Boston (USA)	Clinic	112	80	22	No	Yes	Parent Subject	1) P>C- ADHD 2) P>C (1-year rates)- APD, SUD 3) P>C (lifetime)- APD, Alc, SUD, MDD, BD, AD, etc.
Rasmussen and Gillberg[c]	Gothenburg (Sweden)	Community	55	90	22	Yes	Yes	Subject	1) P>C- ADHD, APD, Alc 2) P=C- SUD, MDD, BD, AD
Weiss and Hechtman[d]	Montreal (Canada)	Clinic	61	59	25	Yes	No	Subject	1) P>C- ADHD symptoms, APD 2) P=C- Alc, SUD, MDD, BD, AD
Mannuzza and Klein[e]	New York (USA)	Clinic	176	85	25	Yes	Yes	Subject	1) P>C- ADHD, APD, SUD 2) P=C- MDD, BD, AD
Klein and Mannuzza[f]	New York (USA)	Clinic	17 P_A, 168 C	–	25	Yes	Yes	Subject	Probands with adult ADHD [P_A] vs. controls [C]- APD: 47 vs. 3%, $p < 0.001$ Alc: 29 vs. 29%, ns SUD: 53 vs. 29%, $p < 0.04$ Mood dis.: 35 vs. 24%, ns MDD: 29 vs. 24%, ns BD: 0 vs. 0% AD: 18 vs. 8%, ns

FU = Follow-up; P = probands, i.e. had ADHD in childhood; C- = controls, i.e. did not have ADHD in childhood; P>C- = probands had significantly higher rates of [X] than controls, P=C- = no significant difference in rates
APD = antisocial personality disorder: MDD = major depressive disorder; BD = bipolar disorder; AD = anxiety disorders; Alc = alcohol abuse or dependence; SUD = SUD other than alcohol; BPD = borderline personality disorder; HPD = histrionic personality disorder; PAPD = passive-aggressive personality disorder; ns = $p > 0.10$.
FU interviewers: psychological assistant supervised by a neuropsychologist in the Barkley & Fischer studies; individuals with undergraduate degrees in psychology in the Biederman study; clinical psychologist and psychiatric social worker in the Klein & Mannuzza studies; psychiatrist in the Rasmussen & Gillberg and Weiss & Hechtman studies.
[a] Barkley et al. [13] and Fischer et al. [14]; [b] Biederman et al. [12]; [c] Rasmussen and Gillberg [15]; [d] Weiss et al. [10]; [e] Mannuzza et al. [16,17]; [f] Unpublished data: of 176 male probands with ADHD in childhood, 17 (10%) reported that ADHD persisted into adulthood, defined as age 18 or older. Rates of various disorders among these 17 male probands with adult ADHD [P_A] are compared to rates among 168 non-ADHD male controls [C].

Table 2. Retrospective studies of adult ADHD

Principal investigator	Sample	n	Mean age years	Interviewer and diagnostic interview	Major findings regarding comorbid adult mental disorders
Studies of adults with ADHD					
Controlled studies					
Biederman[a]	PA- referred adults with ADHD PR- non-referred adult relatives w/ADHD PC- referred children with ADHD CA- comparison adults w/o ADHD	PA- 84 PR- 36 PC- 140 CA- 207	PA- 39 PR- 39 PC- 10 CA- 39	Interviewer not stated Semistructured interview	1) PA>CA- APD, Alc, SUD, MDD, AD 2) PR>CA- APD, Alc, SUD, MDD, AD 3) PA = PR- APD, Alc, SUD, MDD, AD
Biederman[b]	Individuals referred for treatment of adult ADHD (P), and non-referred parents of control children from family genetic studies of ADHD (C)	P- 219 C- 215	P- 38 C- 39	Individuals with undergraduate degrees in psychology Semistructured interview	P>C (lifetime) APD, Alc dependence, SUD, MDD, BD, OCD, GAD, SoP
McGough[c]	Parents of families with 2 children with ADHD- (1) Parents with current ADHD [P]; (2) Parents with no lifetime ADHD [C]	P- 79 C- 283	P- 43 C- 43	'Clinical psychologists or highly trained interviewers with extensive experience' Semistructured interview	P>C- SUD, MDD, BD, 2 or more Ads No rates were reported for APD
Murphy[d]	Individuals w (P) or w/o (C) ADHD referred to an adult ADHD clinic	P- 172 C- 30	P- 32 C- 36	Clinical psychologist Semistructured interview	1) P>C- Alc 2) P=C- SUD, MDD, dysthymia, AD No rates were reported for APD
Murphy[e]	Individuals referred to child & adult ADHD clinics, & community controls	P- 96 C- 64	P- 21 C- 21	Clinical psychologist Unstructured interview	1) P>C- Alc, SUD, dysthymia 2) P=C- APD, MDD, AD
Secnik[f]	Individuals w (P) and w/o (C) adult ADHD as identified from a database of employees of Fortune 200 companies who submitted insurance claims	P- 2,252 C- 2,252	P- 32 C- 32	None: all diagnoses determined from codes entered in the medical database	P>C- APD, Alc or SUD, MDD, BD, AD
Uncontrolled studies					
Downey[g]	Patients treated at an adult ADHD clinic	78	33	A psychiatrist and a clinical psychologist Unstructured interview	) 13% had APD 2) 33% had Alc 3) 21% had SUD 4) 37% had MDD, dysthymia, or depr. disord. NOS 5) 47% had AD or a depressive disorder

Table 2. Continued

Principal investigator	Sample	n	Mean age years	Interviewer and diagnostic interview	Major findings regarding comorbid adult mental disorders
Shekim[h]	Individuals self-referred for treatment of adult ADHD	56	19–65	Interviewer not stated Semistructured interview	1) 34% had Alc 2) 30% had SUD 3) 10% had MDD 4) 25% had dysthymia 5) 25% had cyclothymia 6) 53% had GAD 7) 15% had panic disorder 8) 13% had OCD 9) 8% had phobic disorder No rate was reported for APD
Torgersen[i]	Individuals referred to psychiatric clinics and diagnosed with adult ADHD	45	28	Psychiatrist Unstructured interview	The most common comorbid disorders were: 1) MDD (53% lifetime, 9% current) 2) Cannabis abuse (51% lifetime, 36% current) 3) Amphetamine abuse (49% lifetime, 33% current) 4) Alc (47% lifetime, 33% current) 5) APD (44% lifetime, 0% current)
Studies of individuals with other disorders who were evaluated for adult ADHD					
Substance use disorders					
Clure[j]	Patients treated at three inpatient substance abuse facilities	136	134	Interviewer not stated Semistructured interview	1) 32% had childhood ADHD 2) 49% of above had ADHD into adulthood
Levin[k]	Cocaine abusers treated at outpatient facilities	281	34	The 2 interviewers had an MA & BA in psychology Semistructured interview	1) 12% had childhood ADHD 2) 15% had full or partial adult ADHD 3) 52% of full ADHD had APD

Table 2. Continued

Principal investigator	Sample	n	Mean age years	Interviewer and diagnostic interview	Major findings regarding comorbid adult mental disorders
Schubiner[l]	Randomly selected inpatients from two substance abuse treatment facilities	201	35	Psychology graduate students Semistructured interview	1) 24% had adult ADHD 2) Adult ADHD > no adult ADHD- APD 3) Adult ADHD = no adult ADHD- MDD, BD, GAD, SoP, PTSD
Mood disorders					
Alpert[m]	Patients treated for MDD	116	42	Interviewer not stated Semistructured interview	1) 16% had childhood ADHD 2) 12% had current ADHD
Hesslinger[n]	Patients from an adult ADHD clinic (P_1), and patients from an affective disorders clinic (P_2)	P_1- 40 P_2- 40	P_1- 33 P_2- 36	Psychiatrists Semistructured interview	P_1- 70% had recurrent brief depression P_2- 43% had ADHD
Anxiety disorders					
Adler[o]	Clinic patients with Post-traumatic stress disorder (P) or panic disorder (C)	P- 25 C- 22	P- 60 C- 46	Psychiatrists and a psychologist Semistructured interview	1) P>C- childhood ADHD 2) P=C- current ADHD
Fones[p]	Patients treated for panic disorder	85	36	Interviewer not stated Semistructured interview	1) 24% had full or partial childhood ADHD 2) 65% of above had ADHD into adulthood

P- = ADHD probands, C- = non-ADHD controls; P>C- = probands had significantly higher rates of [X] than controls; P=C- no significant difference in rates.
APD = Antisocial personality disorder, MDD = major depressive disorder, BD = bipolar disorder,
AD = anxiety disorders, OCD = obsessive compulsive disorder, GAD = generalized anxiety disorder, So P= social phobia, PTSD = post-traumatic stress disorder, Alc = alcohol abuse or dependence, SUD = substance use disorder other than alcohol.
[a]Biederman et al. [34]; [b]Biederman et al. [35]; [c]McGough et al. [36]; [d]Murphy and Barkley [37]; [e]Murphy et al. [22]; [f]Secnik et al. [38]; [g]Downey et al. [19]; [h]Shekim et al. [39]; [i]Torgersen et al. [20]; [j]Clure et al. [40]; [k]Levin et al. [41]; [l]Schubiner et al. [21]; [m]Alpert et al. [43]; [n]Hesslinger et al. [42]; [o]Adler et al. [46]; [p]Fones et al. [45].

Another approach to examining the association between ADHD and APD has been to survey groups of incarcerated individuals for the presence of ADHD. Although criminality is not synonymous with APD, the two have considerable overlap. In these groups, rates of ADHD are high. The reliance on retrospective reports from incarcerated individuals is especially problematic, since they may attribute their current legal difficulties to past and current psychopathology. Nevertheless, findings suggest that ADHD is common among incarcerated criminals, probably related to its relationship with APD. However, the methodology in these studies is plagued with difficulties. First, only about half of male prisoners and a fifth of female prisoners have APD [24]. Therefore, drawing conclusions about APD based on prison inmates may be misleading. Second, some investigators (e.g., Abramowitz et al. [25]) report on 'psychopathy,' an overlapping but distinct construct, which hinders interpretation of results. Third, most studies have assessed childhood ADHD, but not its persistence into adulthood [25, 26], thus blurring the distinction between diagnostic and prognostic comorbidity. Fourth, diagnosing the childhood disorder is almost invariably based on retrospective self-reports. Fifth, with few exceptions, diagnoses of childhood ADHD and adult APD or psychopathy are based on cut-off scores on questionnaires completed by prisoners, rather than interviews conducted by experienced clinicians. Finally, failure to take into account comorbid conduct disorder in childhood in predicting later APD precludes interpretation of relationships found with ADHD specifically. Three theories have been proposed to explain the relationship between childhood ADHD and criminality: one is that childhood conduct problems mediate the association (i.e., ADHD alone is insufficient), two is that conduct problems and ADHD are independent predictors, and three, that both are needed to confer increased risk for later antisocial outcomes. All three theories have received some support [27–29]. Nevertheless, results consistently have indicated that both retrospectively reported childhood ADHD and adult ADHD are overrepresented among prison populations (41–67% childhood, 45% in adults), probably, as noted, due to its relationship to APD [30, 31].

In sum, there is evidence suggesting that APD is relatively elevated among adults with ADHD. However, clear interpretation of this relationship requires knowledge of the age of onset of each disorder. If the adults with ADHD and APD had conduct disorder in childhood, whereas others did not, it would indicate consistent diagnostic comorbidity. However, if APD developed later than ADHD, it would argue for prognostic comorbidity. The latter issue is reviewed further on.

Substance Use Disorders

Interest in the comorbidity of adult ADHD and SUDs can be traced back to the 1980s when Wood et al. [32] reported that 33% of their sample of 27 males with alcohol dependence had attention-deficit disorder, residual type (the DSM-III equivalent of adult ADHD). Since then, numerous studies have been published on the prevalence of adult ADHD among substance abusers, most of which have been reviewed by Wilens [33].

Studies have typically targeted alcohol, cannabis, and/or cocaine, since these are among the commonly abused substances in the general population. There is clearly a strong association between substance abuse and dependence with adult ADHD. As shown in table 2, all controlled studies have reported that alcohol, non-alcohol substances, or both are significantly more prevalent among adults with ADHD compared to controls [22, 35–39]. Rates have varied widely (ranging from 20 to 40% for adults with ADHD vs. 5 to 10% for adults without ADHD), depending on the size of the sample, and whether it is abuse or dependence that is reported. Uncontrolled clinical studies have reported that, among adult patients treated for ADHD, one-third have alcohol abuse or dependence, and one-fifth to one-third abuse another substance [19, 20, 39] (see table 2). Finally, both inpatient and outpatient studies of adult substance abusers show relatively high rates of ADHD among these individuals (15–24%) [21, 40, 41] (see table 2). In a study that classified patients by drug of choice (alcohol, cocaine, or both), rates of adult ADHD did not differ [40], leading the authors to conclude that self-medication did not account for the drug use, since the stimulant cocaine was not preferred over alcohol, a central nervous system depressant.

In our prospective follow-up study of children with ADHD, we also found that non-alcohol SUD was significantly more prevalent among those who still had ADHD in adulthood than normal comparisons (53 vs. 29%, $p < 0.04$). In contrast, alcohol abuse/dependence did not differ between adults with continued ADHD and controls (29% for both groups) [23].

The evidence for comorbidity between ADHD and SUD is considerable. Whether it is mediated by another disorder or other factors is not known.

Mood Disorders

Most studies have reported an association between adult ADHD and depressive disorders (major depression, dysthymia, or depressive disorder NOS). Among the six studies of individuals with adult ADHD shown in table 2, only one [37] did not find a relatively higher prevalence of depressive disorder among ADHD adults. Similarly, uncontrolled studies have reported fairly high rates (25–53%) of depressive disorders among individuals with adult ADHD (table 2). Hesslinger et al. [42] reported that 70% of patients in an adult ADHD clinic had recurrent brief depression, whereas 43% of patients seen at a mood disorders clinic had ADHD. Conversely, in a clinic sample of patients with major depression, 12% of patients were judged to have ongoing ADHD [43].

The few controlled studies of bipolar disorder have reported that ADHD adults have an excess of bipolar disorder. Biederman et al. [35] reported rates of 10 vs. 3% ($p < 0.05$), McGough et al. [36] reported 5 vs. 0% ($p < 0.01$), and Secnik et al. [38] reported 4 vs. 1% ($p < 0.01$). In 56 adult patients in a clinic for bipolar patients, Sachs et al. [44] found a 14% rate of childhood ADHD, but do not indicate whether ADHD had persisted through adulthood. Those judged to have had childhood ADHD had earlier bipolar onsets than the non-ADHD bipolar patients. A prevalence of 14% for childhood ADHD seems high, but it does not exceed some population estimates, and does not reinforce the view that ADHD is highly prevalent in bipolar disorder.

In our prospective follow-up study of children with ADHD [16, 17], we did not find that childhood ADHD predicted mood disorders in adulthood, regardless of whether specific mood disorders or a conglomerate category was considered. Rates among probands with adult ADHD and non-ADHD comparisons were as follows: major depressive disorder, 29 vs. 24%, ns; bipolar disorder, 0% in both groups; any mood disorder (MDD, dysthymia, etc.), 35 vs. 24%, ns [23]. Notably, our sample was all male, and ADHD probands were free of conduct disorder in childhood. These two features may be relevant since rates of depression and anxiety disorders are lower in males and conduct disorder in childhood contributes to later risk for these conditions. In addition, the number of adults with ADHD was relatively small, and would not provide power to detect an infrequent outcome, such as bipolar disorder.

Anxiety Disorders

In the case of anxiety disorders, findings are inconsistent. Some controlled studies report elevated rates in ADHD in adults [34–36, 38], whereas others do not [22, 37]. Fones et al. [45] reported that 15% of patients with panic disorder had adult ADHD. As with other studies of this kind, the lack of a comparison group is problematic. In addition, the authors do not state who conducted the evaluations, and whether these individuals were blind to study hypotheses. In a small, non-blinded study, the rate of adult ADHD did not differ between patients with panic disorder and those with post-traumatic stress disorder [46]. In our prospective adult follow-up study of boys with ADHD [16, 17], there was no significant preponderance of anxiety disorders in adulthood among probands with adult ADHD compared to non-ADHD controls (18 vs. 8%, ns). In conclusion, a relationship between adult ADHD and anxiety disorders is not established, and requires further systematic study.

Comorbidity in Adults with ADHD in the General Population

All the above studies, whether cross-sectional or of psychiatric disorders longitudinal, have dealt with clinical cases of ADHD. It is well known that comorbidity is higher in clinical than population samples. Only one recent US population study has reported on comorbidity in adults with ADHD [47]. It estimated the prevalence of ADHD to be 4.4% in 18- to 44-year-olds. Comorbidity rates were significantly elevated in this group compared to adults without ADHD. Respective rates were: mood disorders 38 and 11% ($p < 0.05$); anxiety disorders, 47 and 19% ($p < 0.05$); SUD, 15 and 6% ($p < 0.05$), and intermittent explosive disorder, 29 and 6% ($p < 0.05$). Among the mood and anxiety disorders, all the individual component disorders were significantly elevated in the ADHD adults. Not so in the case of SUDs – only drug dependence was significantly higher in the adults with ADHD (4.4 vs. 0.6%, $p < 0.05$). There were no significant differences in alcohol abuse, alcohol dependence, and drug abuse. APD was not addressed in the report. Surprisingly, relative comorbidity rates are not appreciably different from those reported in clinical studies. Inevitably, the study suffers from limitations inherent in retrospective studies that rely on self-reports exclusively, where the positive predictive value of ADHD diagnoses in childhood is likely to be poor.

Factors Influencing Diagnostic Comorbidity

ADHD is more prevalent in men than women, prompting conjecture about possible differences in the disorder and its course between the two sexes. The evidence suggests that men and women have similar comorbidity. The Boston group reported that comorbidity did not differ between men and women [48], and also found no difference in comorbidity between referred and non-referred adults with ADHD [35] (table 2). No other factors have been examined, and little is known about factors that influence diagnostic comorbidity.

Prognostic Comorbidity of Childhood ADHD

Prognostic comorbidity requires two conditions. One, the index disorder (in this case ADHD) must precede the comorbid disorder. Two, the index condition must remain active during the development of the later condition. If the index disorder remits, but predicts other conditions, the index disorder represents a risk factor for subsequent pathology, but strictly speaking, the index and other disorder are not comorbid. This type of information is limited in the case of ADHD. It requires that comprehensive diagnostic information be obtained about all major psychiatric disorders in childhood. In some cases, the absence of comorbidity with childhood ADHD can be taken for granted. SUDs and contact with judicial system (e.g., arrests, convictions and incarcerations) are, for all practical purposes, non-existent in children. However, such is not the case for a host of other conditions. Conduct disorder, for one, has been shown to be highly comorbid with childhood ADHD and strongly predictive of APD [49].

To date, there has been no adult longitudinal follow-up of children with ADHD that can report on the incidence (new onsets) of a variety of psychiatric disorders. This is critical since, as noted, childhood ADHD is highly comorbid with a number of disorders, especially conduct disorder, and anxiety and mood disorders [50]. For example, major depression has been diagnosed in as many as 75% of children, and anxiety disorders in about 30%. Consequently, their comorbid presence in adults with ADHD cannot be attributed unequivocally to the prognostic comorbidity of childhood ADHD. As we note above, substance use and abuse are not features of preadolescents; therefore, outcomes from studies that have followed preadolescents could not have been affected by the presence of these conditions in childhood. The same is not true of longitudinal studies that include adolescents (e.g., the Boston studies).

The Boston group [12] reported a 10-year follow-up of a cohort of 6- to 18-year-olds with ADHD compared to non-ADHD comparisons (mean age 21 at follow-up).

This is the only longitudinal study that controls for initial comorbidity. The report illustrates the potential confound of initial comorbidity in follow-up studies. Initial comorbidity rates were: for major depression, 29%; anxiety disorders, 44%, and conduct disorder, 21%. After controlling for initial comorbidity and relevant baseline characteristics, the study found no difference in 1-year rates of major depression, bipolar disorder, or anxiety disorders between the ADHD and control groups. Only APDs and nicotine dependence were significantly elevated in ADHD probands. Unfortunately, the relationships between initial and outcome comorbidity are not presented. Although the stated goal of the study was to inform on the adult outcome of ADHD, the mean age was just 21, and the sample at follow-up included adolescents. Furthermore, the inclusion of a wide age range confounds interpretation since those diagnosed at 17 are likely to represent a different population of children with ADHD from those identified at age 6. In the latter group, a substantial proportion will no longer have ADHD at age 17. Finally, although 58% of the original ADHD sample no longer met criteria for ADHD at the 10-year mark, the authors do not indicate the distribution of comorbid disorders in the remitted versus persisted ADHD cases, limiting our understanding of the findings.

In the New York follow-up study of children with ADHD, conduct disorder was systematically excluded since the clinical trials then under way required that children have 'uncomplicated' ADHD. No other sample of ADHD children provides the opportunity to determine whether ADHD alone predicts the development of antisocial disorder. In two independent samples of children with ADHD, but no conduct disorder (mean age 8 years; range 6–12), we found that the development of antisocial disorder was much more frequent in probands than non-ADHD-matched peers. At mean age 18, APD was ongoing in 37% of probands versus 3% in controls [51, 52]. At average age 25, respective rates were 15 and 2% [16, 17]. In adolescence, the excess of APD was completely accounted for by probands who had retained ADHD. The prevalence of comorbid antisocial disorder among persistent ADHD cases was 48%, as opposed to 17% in probands whose ADHD had remitted, no different from controls (8%). These findings reflect prognostic comorbidity of ADHD for APD in adolescence. In adulthood, we found that probands who retained ADHD beyond age 18 had significantly higher rates of APD than those who remitted before age 18 (47 vs. 23%, $p = 0.03$). However, unlike adolescence, the excess of APD in the adults was no longer restricted to those who still had ADHD. APD had developed functional autonomy. Of relevance, in this study, in virtually all instances, the age of onset for APD preceded the age at which SUD began [51], thus pointing to a cascading developmental trajectory from ADHD to APD, and then SUD.

Relatedly, we found that criminal behavior was more frequent in ADHD probands at the average age of 22 than in controls [53]. Respective rates were: arrests 39 and 20% ($p < 0.02$); convictions 28 and 11% ($p < 0.01$), and incarcerations, 9 and 1% ($p < 0.05$). These negative judicial outcomes were completely accounted for by the presence of APD. In other words, the rates of criminality did not differ between probands without

APD and controls, even among probands who still had ADHD. Thus, ADHD alone does not predict criminality; the latter requires the development of APD. Similar differences in criminality between probands and controls were found at age 38. Relying on judicial records of probands and controls in New York State, respective rates were: arrests 47 and 24% ($p < 0.01$); convictions 42 and 14% ($p < 0.002$); incarcerations, and 15 and 1% ($p < 0.02$). A history of APD or SUDs was an independent predictor of multiple arrests in probands [23].

Although the New York study excluded ADHD children with conduct disorders, oppositional defiant disorder was allowed. It is therefore possible that the oppositional defiant disorder contributed to the development of APD, rather than ADHD itself. Such was not the case. Oppositional defiant disorder symptoms were not associated with the maintenance of ADHD, or with the development of APD [54]. In sum, childhood ADHD is a precursor of adolescent onset APD, especially in those who retain ADHD, even in the absence of comorbid oppositional defiant disorder or conduct disorder in childhood.

As noted above, SUDs have been found to be relatively more frequent in children with ADHD followed into adulthood. The question here is whether this excess is limited to those who retain ADHD, as in the case of APD. In the New York study, the only report thus far to address this issue, the development of SUDs was not a function of retention of ADHD (53 vs. 45% in persistent and remitted ADHD). Probands who retained ADHD but had not developed APD did not differ from controls with respect to SUDs. Thus, we did not find prognostic comorbidity of ADHD for SUDs. Rather, ADHD represents a risk factor through the mediation of APD. There did not appear to be differential prevalence of anxiety and mood disorders in cases who had retained ADHD into adulthood and those in whom it desisted, but the number of subjects with persistent ADHD is small (rates of mood disorders, 35 vs. 22%, anxiety disorders, 18 vs. 18%, ns).

There would be great merit in understanding factors that influence the prognostic comorbidity of ADHD. To do so requires the identification of characteristics that predict the maintenance of ADHD into adulthood. Efforts in this direction have been disappointing and no consistent evidence points to patterns of predictive value for any feature [55]. One study reports that severity of childhood ADHD and treatment for ADHD predicted persistence into adulthood [56]. However, these reports were retrospectively obtained from adults, and current status may have influenced recall. Neuroimaging work in progress aiming at distinguishing genetic characteristics among ADHD children with good versus poor outcomes may be generating promising results [57].

Summary and Conclusions

Prospective follow-up studies of children with ADHD have provided limited information regarding diagnostic comorbidity among individuals with adult ADHD. Few studies have reported rates of comorbid disorders among unremitted and remitted cases of ADHD (table 1). Our findings indicate that ADHD leads to the development of APD even in the absence of conduct disorder in childhood. In turn, APD fosters the development of SUDs. Thus, there appears to be no direct relationship between persistent ADHD and SUDs. Despite diverse methodologies across clinical studies of adults with ADHD (tables 1, 2), reports of elevated rates of APD and SUDs are consistent. In contrast, reports of depressive and anxiety disorders are variable. Relative rates may vary with type of clinical sample (inpatient, outpatient), type of assessment (unstructured and semistructured clinical interviews and highly structured inquiry), evaluator (clinician, lay interviewer), and sample characteristics such as socioeconomic status that affect rates of APD.

Acknowledgement

The authors thank Jonathan Avery for his assistance.

References

1 Feinstein AR: The pre-therapeutic classification of co-morbidity in chronic disease. J Chron Dis 1970; 23:455–468.

2 Kaplan MH, Feinstein AR: The importance of classifying initial co-morbidity in evaluating the outcome of diabetes mellitus. J Chron Dis 1974;27: 387–404.

3 Fyer AJ, Liebowitz MR, Klein DF: Treatment trials, comorbidity, and syndromal complexity; in Maser JD, Cloninger CR (eds): Comorbidity of Mood and Anxiety Disorders. Washington, American Psychiatric Press, 1990, pp 669–679.

4 Kraemer HC, Wilson KA, Hayward C: Lifetime prevalence and pseudocomorbidity in psychiatric research. Arch Gen Psychiatry 2006;63:604–608.

5 Milliberger S, Biederman J, Faraone SV, Murphy J, Tsuang MT: Attention-deficit hyperactivity disorder and comorbid disorders: issues of overlapping symptoms. Am J Psychiatry 1995;152:1793–1799.

6 American Psychiatric Association: Diagnostic and Statistical Manual of Mental Disorders, Text Revision, ed 4 (DSM-IV-TR). Washington, APA, 2000.

7 March JS, Swanson JM, Arnold LE, Hoza B, Conners CK, Hinshaw S, Hechtman L, Kraemer HC, Greenhill LL, Abikoff H, Elliott G, Jensen PS, Newcorn JH, Vitiello B, Newcorn J, Severe JB, Wells KC, Pelham WE: Anxiety as a predictor and outcome variable in the multimodal treatment study of children with ADHD. J Abnorm Child Psychol 2000;28:527–541.

8 Mannuzza S, Klein RG, Klein DF, Bessler A, Shrout P: Accuracy of adult recall of childhood attention-deficit hyperactivity disorder. Am J Psychiatry 2002; 159:1882–1888.

9 Fleiss JL, William JBW, Dubro AF: The logistic regression of psychiatric data. J Psychiatr Res 1986; 20:195–209.

10 Weiss G, Hechtman L, Milroy T, Perlman T: Psychiatric status of hyperactives as adults. J Am Acad Child Adolesc Psychiatry 1985;24:211–220.

11 Cox A, Rutter M, Yule B, Quinton D: Bias resulting from missing information. Br J Prev Soc Med 1977; 31:131–136.

12 Biederman J, Monuteaux MC, Mick E, Spencer T, Wilens TE, Silva JM, Snyder LE, Faraone SV: Young adult outcome of attention-deficit hyperactivity disorder: a controlled 10-year follow-up study. Psychol Med 2006;36:167–179.

13 Barkley RA, Fischer M, Smallish L, Fletcher K: The persistence of attention-deficit/hyperactivity disorder into young adulthood as a function of reporting source and definition of disorder. J Abnorm Psychol 2002;111:279–289.

14 Fischer M, Barkley RA, Smallish L, Fletcher K: Young adult follow-up of hyperactive children: self-reported psychiatric disorders, comorbidity, and the role of childhood conduct problems and teen CD. J Abnorm Child Psychol 2002;30:463–475.

15 Rasmussen P, Gillberg C: Natural outcome of ADHD with developmental coordination disorder at age 22 years: a controlled, longitudinal, community-based study. J Am Acad Child Adolesc Psychiatry 2000;39:1424–1431.
16 Mannuzza S, Klein RG, Bessler A, Malloy P, LaPadula M: Adult outcome of hyperactive boys: educational achievement, occupational rank, and psychiatric status. Arch Gen Psychiatry 1993;50:565–576.
17 Mannuzza S, Klein RG, Bessler A, Malloy P, La Padula M: Adult psychiatric status of hyperactive boys grown up. Am J Psychiatry 1998;155:493–498.
18 Mannuzza S, Klein RG, Moulton JL III: Persistence of attention-deficit hyperactivity disorder into adulthood: what have we learned from the prospective follow-up studies? J Atten Disord 2003;7:93–100.
19 Downey KK, Stelson FW, Pomerleau OF, Giordani B: Adult attention-deficit hyperactivity disorder: psychological test profiles in a clinical population. J Nerv Ment Dis 1997;185:32–38.
20 Torgersen T, Gjervan B, Rasmussen K: ADHD in adults: a study of clinical characteristics, impairment and comorbidity. Nord J Psychiatry 2006;60: 38–43.
21 Schubiner H, Tzelepis A, Milberger S, Lockhart N, Kruger M, Kelley BJ, Schoener EP: Prevalence of attention-deficit/hyperactivity disorder and conduct disorder among substance abusers. J Clin Psychiatry 2000;61:244–251.
22 Murphy KR, Barkley RA, Bush T: Young adults with attention-deficit hyperactivity disorder: subtype differences in comorbidity, educational, and clinical history. J Nerv Ment Dis 2002;190:147–157.
23 Klein R, Mannuzza S, Castellanos FX: Aging aspects of ADHD. Paper presented at the 2nd International Congress of ADHD, May 20, 2009.
24 Fazel S, Danesh J: Serious mental disorder in 23,000 prisoners: a systematic review of 62 surveys. Lancet 2002;359:545–550.
25 Abramowitz CS, Kosson DS, Seidenberg M: The relationship between childhood attention-deficit hyperactivity disorder and conduct problems and adult psychopathy in male inmates. Pers Individ Diff 2004;36:1031–1047.
26 Johansson P, Kerr M, Andershed H: Linking adult psychopathy with childhood hyperactivity-impulsivity-attention problems and conduct problems through retrospective self-reports. J Pers Disord 2005;19:94–101.
27 Babinski LM, Hartsough CS, Lambert NM: Childhood conduct problems, hyperactivity-impulsivity, and inattention as predictors of adult criminal activity. J Child Psychiatry Psychol 1999;40: 347–355.
28 Lilienfeld SO, Waldman ID: The relationship between childhood attention-deficit hyperactivity disorder and adult antisocial behavior reexamined: the problem of heterogeneity. Clin Psychol Rev 1990;10:699–725.
29 Lynam DR: Early identification of chronic offenders: Who is the fledgling psychopath? Psychol Bull 1996;120:209–234.
30 Rösler M, Retz W, Retz-Junginger P, Hengesch G, Schneider M, Supprian T, Schwitzgebel P, Pinhard K, Dovi-Akue N, Wender P, Thome J: Prevalence of attention-deficit/hyperactivity disorder and comorbid disorders in young male prison inmates. Eur Arch Psychiatry Clin Neurosci 2004;254:365–371.
31 Vitelli R: Prevalence of childhood conduct and attention-deficit hyperactivity disorders in adult maximum-security inmates. Int J Offender Ther Comp Criminol 1996;40:263–271.
32 Wood D, Wender PH, Reimherr FW: The prevalence of attention-deficit disorder, residual type, or minimal brain dysfunction, in a population of male alcoholic patients. Am J Psychiatry 1983;140;95–98.
33 Wilens TE: Attention-deficit/hyperactivity disorder and the substance use disorders: the nature of the relationship, subtypes at risk, and treatment issues. Psychiatr Clin North Am 2004;27:283–301.
34 Biederman J, Faraone SV, Spencer T, Wilens T, Norman D, Lapey KA, Mick E, Lehman BK, Doyle A: Patterns of psychiatric comorbidity, cognition, and psychosocial functioning in adults with attention-deficit hyperactivity disorder. Am J Psychiatry 1993;150:1792–1798.
35 Biederman J, Faraone SV, Monuteaux MC, Bober M, Cadogen E: Gender effects on attention-deficit/ hyperactivity disorder in adults, revisited. Biol Psychiatry 2004;55:692–700.
36 McGough JJ, Smalley SL, McCracken JT, Yang M, Del'Homme M, Lynn DE, Loo S: Psychiatric comorbidity in adult attention-deficit hyperactivity disorder: findings from multiplex families. Am J Psychiatry 2005;162:1621–1627.
37 Murphy K, Barkley RA: Attention-deficit hyperactivity disorder in adults: Comorbidities and adaptive impairments. Compr Psychiatry 1996;37: 393–401.
38 Secnik K, Swensen A, Lage MJ: Comorbidities and costs of adult patients diagnosed with attention-deficit hyperactivity disorder. Pharmacoeconomics 2005;23:93–102.
39 Shekim WO, Asarnow RF, Hess E, Zaucha K, Wheeler N: A clinical and demographic profile of a sample of adults with attention-deficit hyperactivity disorder, residual state. Compr Psychiatry 1990;31: 416–425.

40 Clure C, Brady KT, Saladin ME, Johnson D, Waid R, Rittenbury M: Attention-deficit/hyperactivity disorder and substance use: symptom pattern and drug choice. Am J Drug Alcohol Abuse 1999;25:441–448.
41 Levin FR, Evans SM, Kleber HD: Prevalence of adult attention-deficit/hyperactivity disorder among cocaine abusers seeking treatment. Drug Alcohol Depend 1998;52:15–25.
42 Hesslinger B, van Elst LT, Mochan F, Ebert D: A psychopathological study into the relationship between attention-deficit hyperactivity disorder in adult patients and recurrent brief depression. Acta Physiol Scand 2003;107:385–389.
43 Alpert JE, Maddocks A, Nierenberg AA, O'Sullivan R, Pava JA, Worthington JJ III, Biederman J, Rosenbaum JF, Fava M: Attention-deficit hyperactivity disorder in childhood among adults with major depression. Psychiatry Res 1996;62:213–219.
44 Sachs GS, Baldassano CF, Truman CJ, Guille C: Comorbidity of attention-deficit hyperactivity disorder with early- and late-onset bipolar disorder. Am J Psychiatry 2000;157:466–468.
45 Fones CSL, Pollack MH, Susswein L, Otto M: History of childhood attention-deficit hyperactivity disorder features among adults with panic disorder. J Affect Disord 2000;58:99–106.
46 Kessler RC, Adler L, Barkley R, Biederman J, Conner CK, Demler O, Faraone SV, Greenhill LL, Howes MJ: The prevalence and correlates of adult ADHD in the United States: results from the national comorbidity survey replication. Am J Psychiatry 2006;163:716–723.
47 Adler LA, Kunz M, Chua HC, Rotrosen J, Resnick SG: Attention-deficit/hyperactivity disorder in adult patients with posttraumatic stress disorder: Is ADHD a vulnerability factor? J Attn Disord 2004;8:11–16.
48 Biederman J, Faraone SV, Spencer T, Wilens T, Mick E, Lapey KA: Gender differences in a sample of adults with attention-deficit hyperactivity disorder. Psychiatry Res 1994;53:13–29.
49 Robins LN: Deviant Children Grown Up. Baltimore, Williams & Wilkins, 1966.
50 Spencer TJ: ADHD and comorbidity in childhood. J Clin Psychiatry 2006;67:27–31.
51 Gittelman R, Mannuzza S, Shenker R, Bonagura N: Hyperactive boys almost grown up. I. Psychiatric status. Arch Gen Psychiatry 1985;42:937–947.
52 Mannuzza S, Klein RG, Bonagura N, Malloy P, Giampino TL, Addalli KA: Hyperactive boys almost grown up. V. Replication of psychiatric status. Arch Gen Psychiatry 1991;48:77–83.
53 Mannuzza S, Klein RG, Konig PH, Giampino TL: Hyperactive boys almost grown up. IV. Criminality and its relationship to psychiatric status. Arch Gen Psychiatry 1989;46:1073–1079.
54 Mannuzza S, Klein RG, Abikoff H, Moulton JL III: Significance of childhood conduct problems to later development of conduct disorder among children with ADHD: a prospective follow-up study. J Abnorm Child Psychol 2004;32:565–573.
55 Mannuzza S, Klein RG: Predictors of outcome of children with attention-deficit hyperactivity disorder. Child Adolesc Psychiatr Clin N Am 1992;1:567–578.
56 Kessler RC, Adler LA, Barkley R, Biederman J, Conners CK, Faraone SV, Greenhill LL, Jaeger S, Secnik K, Spencer T, Ustun TB, Zaslavsky AM: Patterns and predictors of attention-deficit/hyperactivity disorder persistence into adulthood: results from the national comorbidity survey replication. Biol Psychiatry 2005;57:1442–1451.
57 Shaw P, Gornick M, Lerch J, Addigton A, Seal J, Greenstein D, Sharp W, Evans A, Giedd JN, Castellanos FX, Rapoport JL: Polymorphisms of the dopamine D4 receptor, clinical outcome, and cortical structure in attention-deficit/hyperactivity disorder. Arch Gen Psychiatry 2007;64:921–931.

Prof. Rachel G. Klein, PhD
Department of Child and Adolescent Psychiatry, New York University School of Medicine
New York University Child Study Center, Floor 13
215 Lexington Avenue
New York, NY 10016 (USA)
Tel. +1 212 263 8389, Fax +1 212 263 3691, E-Mail rachel.klein@med.nyu.edu

Retz W, Klein RG (eds): Attention-Deficit Hyperactivity Disorder (ADHD) in Adults.
Key Issues in Mental Health. Basel, Karger, 2010, vol 176, pp 144–158

Adult Attention-Deficit Hyperactivity Disorder – Functional Impairment, Conduct Problems and Criminality

Michael Rösler

Neurocentre, Saarland University Hospital, Institute for Forensic Psychology and Psychiatry, Homburg/Saar, Germany

Abstract

Attention-deficit hyperactivity disorder (ADHD) is very frequent in offender populations. 'Pure' ADHD seldom occurs in these persons. The majority of individuals suffer from ADHD in combination with conduct disorder. The risk of developing antisocial and delinquent behavior during later life is mediated by childhood or adolescent-onset conduct problems and not by ADHD itself. Persons suffering from ADHD without conduct disorder do not have an elevated risk for the development of delinquency. The comparison of offenders or persons with conduct problems with and without ADHD reveals that ADHD has modulating effects on the psychopathology and on the structure as well as the course of delinquent behavior. A general impact of ADHD can be separated from specific modulation factors. Regarding general influences, there is growing evidence that offenders with ADHD start their criminal career earlier than those without ADHD. Moreover, the risk of committing recidivistic crimes is significantly higher in offenders with ADHD. A further general finding is the declining prevalence of ADHD with age. A specific finding is that the prevalence of ADHD is not on the same level in different forms of crime. ADHD is very common in sexual and violent offenders. On the contrary, ADHD is uncommon in offenders who commit fraud. Regarding violent behavior, persons with ADHD tend to commit reactive violence while offenders without ADHD preferentially display proactive violence. Offenders with ADHD have slightly increased psychopathic traits but they do not score in the range of typical psychopathy according to Hare. The psychopathology of ADHD and that of psychopathy are two different concepts which show no considerable overlap.

Attention-deficit hyperactivity disorder (ADHD) is a chronic disorder which can be diagnosed in early childhood. The disorder usually persists during adolescence and in 60% of the affected persons the psychopathology is partially or fully present in adulthood. The transnational prevalence in adulthood is 3.4% [1]. In the USA the prevalence of adult ADHD is 4.4% according to the National Comorbidity Survey [2]. In Germany, a prevalence of 3.1% was found [1]. Due to developmental factors in adult life the psychopathology might be somewhat different as compared with earlier life: inattention, hyperactivity and impulsivity is the classical triad at all life stages while disorganization, hot temper, stress intolerance and affective or emotional lability might be typical psychopathological features associated with adult ADHD [3–7].

ADHD is associated in many cases with considerable risks regarding daily functioning and social adaptation [8]. Moreover, ADHD has found growing interest in forensic psychiatry due to the observation that 20–25% of the children and adolescents affected with ADHD display antisocial personality disorder (APD) during adult life [9–11]. Persons with APD are a core population in forensic psychiatric and offender samples. A further point of interest is the increased prevalence of ADHD in offender populations.

Dysfunction in Activities of Daily Living

As compared with their intellectual capability, the number of high-quality graduations at school or regarding vocational education is decreased. Individuals suffering from ADHD are thought to be underachievers in many cases. They have an increased number of classroom suspensions and school exclusions. They have a higher risk of being fired and the number of jobs in a given time period is increased. The rate of conflicts with colleagues and supervisors is relatively high [8]. Times of unemployment are not rare.

They start sexual activities significantly earlier compared with adolescents without ADHD. The risk of sexually-transmitted disorders is much higher as well as unwanted pregnancies [12]. Affected individuals describe their marital and family situation less favorably as persons without ADHD. Separation and divorce rates are significantly increased. Many adults with ADHD have difficulties with parenting skills.

The risk of accidents at home, school, and vocational affairs or during leisure activities is much higher than in controls. Even in cases of severe accidental injury, ADHD is significantly overrepresented [13, 14].

The risk of violations of road traffic rules in adults with ADHD is much higher. The prevalence of accidents is increased, as well as driving under the influence of alcohol, driving without a driving license and speeding [15].

ADHD and Criminality

General Factors

There is no doubt that the prevalence of ADHD in forensic and criminological populations is much higher when compared with the general population. According to a survey of the available studies in adolescents by Vermeiren et al. [16], the prevalence

Table 1. Prevalence of ADHD in different offender populations [modified according to 16]

Author	n	Country	Results
Hollander and Turner [57]	185	USA	19% developmental abnormalities with and without ADHD
Milin et al. [58]	111	Canada	19% ADD (23% A, 24% H, 33% I)
Haapasalo and Hamalainen [59]	89	Finland	50% ADHD
Richards [60]	100	Australia	4% ADHD
Timmons-Mitchell et al. [17]	50	USA	72% ADHD male: 76%, female 68%
Ulzen and Hamilton [18]	98	Canada	27% (controls 2%, male 29%, female 18%)
Doreleijers et al. [61]	108	Netherlands	14% ADHD
Pliszka et al. [62]	50	USA	18% ADHD
Vermeiren et al. [63]	72	Belgium	19% ADHD
Ruchkin et al. [64]	358	Russia	18% lifetime, 3% cross-section
Rösler et al. [19]	129	Germany	Males: 45% ADHD (DSM-IV)
Rösler et al. [31]	110	Germany	Females: 10% ADHD (DSM-IV)

of ADHD in offender populations may vary between 4 and 72%. In numerous studies it has been found that both male and female delinquent populations display high prevalence rates of ADHD [17, 18]. The broad range of results emerging from the studies listed in table 1 chiefly arises from very different study populations in countries with different criminal law systems. Nevertheless, many of the cited studies estimate ADHD prevalence between 14 and 19%. In a German study with 129 male adolescent and young adult prison inmates, the prevalence of full clinical pictures of ADHD according to DSM-IV was 45% [19].

It has to be pointed out that in offender populations 'pure' ADHD was very rare. In almost all cases, ADHD is associated with comorbid conduct disorder (CD). This is a specific combination which can be diagnosed according to ICD-10 as a hyperkinetic disorder of social behavior (F90.1). According to DSM-IV, a diagnostic category like this is still lacking. The differentiation between ADHD and ADHD with CD is very important because it is essential to know whether dysfunctional and social problems or even criminal behavior can be linked to ADHD, CD, or to both disorders.

After a long and divergent discussion it became more and more evident that the risk for the development of criminal behavior in persons suffering from ADHD is mediated predominantly by comorbid CD. Babinski et al. [20] found that conduct problems and hyperactivity/impulsivity but not inattention contributed to the risk of criminal involvement in a group of offenders with recidivistic crimes. On the other hand the vast majority of studies indicated that CD and not ADHD predicts adult antisociality. These authors did not find an independent effect of ADHD on antisociality and argued that CD is the main risk factor for antisocial and criminal behavior [21–24]. Only few researchers reported findings supporting the notion that ADHD may contribute independently from CD to the risk of later criminality [25, 26]. Today we are in the position to sum up by saying that CD is the main risk factor for later criminality, especially for severe criminal acts, while individuals with ADHD alone may have only an increased risk for minor delinquency like traffic violations or misdemeanors but not for felony crimes. In the given context the question arises: What are the critical developmental periods in which the risk behavior can be detected?

Follow-up studies with children suffering from ADHD and CD revealed high rates of APD in later life [9, 27, 28]. Interestingly, a significant proportion of ADHD children without CD at the time of inclusion in the New York follow-up studies [10] were diagnosed with APD in later life, suggesting that early-onset CD is not a necessary condition for adult APD. Thus it is possible to differentiate two forms of ADHD associated with CD: ADHD with childhood-onset CD and ADHD with adolescent-onset CD (fig. 1).

In the majority of cases, CD is present before the age of 10 years indicating a risk for later antisociality and criminal behavior. In a smaller but significant proportion, conduct problems appear during adolescence. Like early-onset CD this constellation can lead to later criminality [29]. At present it is not definitely clear whether ADHD with childhood- or adolescent-onset CD differ in terms of their course during adult life. Nevertheless, there is evidence that ADHD with childhood-onset CD tends more to a chronic course whereas ADHD with adolescent-onset CD may have an episodic character [30].

ADHD-Specific Findings

Prevalence of ADHD

The model that the risk for later antisociality and criminality in individuals with ADHD is not mediated by ADHD itself but by associated CD does not exclude the possibility that ADHD may have a modulating effect on the course of the antisocial or criminal behavior and other interesting forensic variables. Thus it is necessary to compare individuals suffering from APD with and without ADHD as well as offender populations with and without ADHD. Interestingly, there is an age-dependent decline of the prevalence of ADHD in forensic and offender populations. Satterfield et al. [23] published the results of a 30-year prospective follow-up study of hyperactive boys with CD and found that there was a steady decline in offending rates with increasing age. The mean age of desistance was 30 years. In a study with 110 incarcerated women [31], we divided the population into three groups in accordance to their age. The first group comprised all individuals with an age up to 25 years and the second group consisted of all women with an age between 26 and 45 years. In the third group were patients older than 45 years. Among the first group with young females

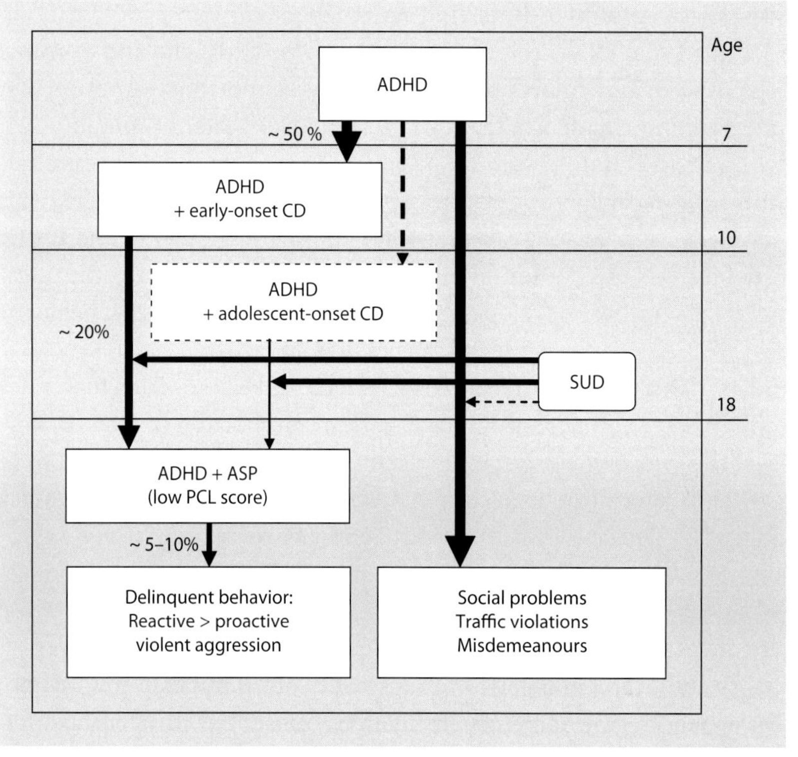

Fig. 1. Developmental pathways from early childhood ADHD to adult ADHD with and without antisociality and criminal behavior. The percent specifications declare how many individuals from the initial childhood population arrive at the endpoint. SUD = Substance use disorder [according to 65].

the prevalence of ADHD according to DSM-IV was around 18% and in the second group the prevalence was 10%. Among the third group, no patient with a full clinical picture of ADHD was found.

Furthermore, we analyzed a population of 595 male offenders who were admitted consecutively to our facility for a forensic psychiatric evaluation [Rösler and Retz, unpubl. data]. Nearly one-half of the individuals were incarcerated. All types of offences from simple misdemeanors to severe felony crimes were present. The prevalence of ADHD in the first group (until 25 years) was 23.2%. The second group (26–50 years) displayed a prevalence of 9.2% and in the next two groups (51–75 years, 76 years and more) prevalence rates further declined to 5 and 5.3%, respectively, providing further evidence that age clearly affects the prevalence of ADHD in male and female offender populations (fig. 2).

These data support the notion that ADHD is significantly overrepresented in adolescent and young adult offender populations, but with advancing age the prevalence tends towards normal.

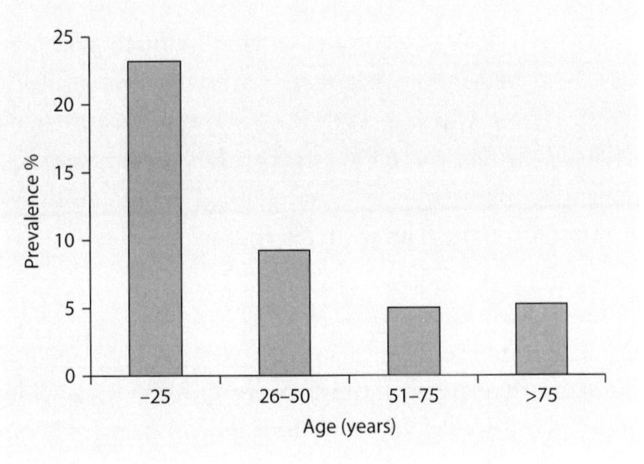

Fig. 2. Age-dependent prevalence of ADHD. 595 male offenders under forensic psychiatric evaluation. The population has committed all types of crimes from misdemeanors to severe felony crimes.

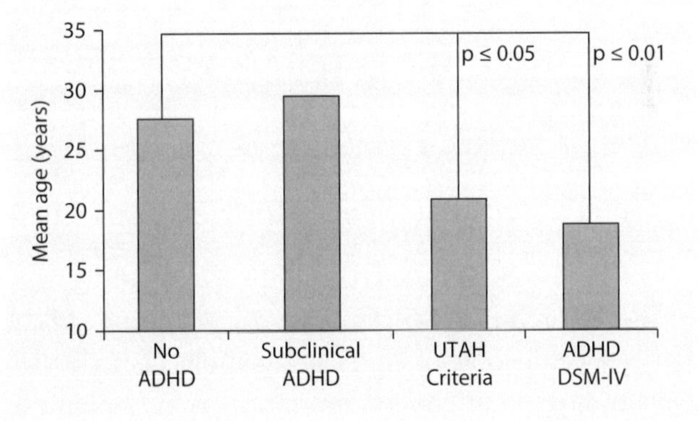

Fig. 3. Age at first conviction in 110 incarcerated women. The ADHD diagnosis was made according to DSM-IV and to the Utah criteria [3]. Subclinical cases fulfilled in earlier life the DSM-IV criteria and had a partial remission of psychopathology thereafter.

Age of First Conviction

In our study [19] with incarcerated young men with CD the age at first conviction was 15.5 years, when ADHD was present. In the group with CD but without ADHD the age at first conviction was 17.5 years. More than 51% of individuals with ADHD had committed crimes before the age of 14 years compared with 27% of those without ADHD. In a later study with 110 incarcerated women, the age of first conviction was 9 years earlier in the ADHD group as compared with women without ADHD [31]. This finding is presented in figure 3. Similar findings were reported earlier by Loeber et al. [21], Moffitt [30, 32] and Ziegler et al. [33].

Recidivistic Criminality

In a study by Ziegler et al. [33] an association between the current diagnosis of ADHD in incarcerated adult male offenders and previous delinquency was found.

The odds ratio (OR) to be a recidivistic offender was 3.8 (95% CI 2.0–7.1) in the presence of ADHD as compared with individuals without ADHD. A similar association was described by Blocher et al. [34], who had examined 127 sexual offenders. From the subgroup without ADHD, 27.4% had had earlier convictions for sexual crimes, whereas the rate was 64.3% in the ADHD subgroup (OR 4.8, 95% CI 1.5–15.3). These findings support the view that delinquency in adults with ADHD refers not to single events arising from an individual's normal life.

Family Transmission of Criminality and Other Social Parameters

In our study with adolescent and young adult incarcerated men, we found significantly more relatives in the families of individuals with ADHD and CD who had been imprisoned due to severe crimes as compared with offenders suffering solely from CD but not from ADHD [19]. Other socio-psychiatric parameters like vocational education, unemployment rate or robust partnerships did not differ between the two populations.

In a female offender population, more problems with the social surrounding were present in individuals with ADHD as compared with those without ADHD [31].

Type of Offence

Babinski et al. [20] suggested that persons with ADHD may be at higher risk for less severe crimes, whereas individuals with CD are at higher risk for severe criminal activities such as robbery or assault.

The prevalence of ADHD in different offender types is not distributed equally. In earlier research [33] we examined the prevalence of childhood ADHD psychopathology in specific male offender populations. The prevalence of childhood ADHD psychopathology in offenders committing fraud did not differ from controls. Individuals who had committed property crimes had slightly increased childhood ADHD. The highest prevalence rates were found in populations with sexual crime. The study by Blocher et al. [34] concerning sexual delinquency found a cross-sectional diagnosis of current ADHD of about 28%. Interestingly there was no difference in ADHD between the three main offender groups: rape, sexual abuse of children, and exhibitionism. In a recent study we found evidence that there is only small increase in the prevalence of ADHD with regard to different violent offender populations, if the populations were classified according to the criminal code [35]. Apparently the clustering of offenders in terms of the offences by the rules of the criminal law is too heterogeneous and does not allow for precise investigations.

The construct of a dichotomy between reactive-impulsive and affective violence and a proactive-predatory and instrumental violence [36, 37] offers the opportunity to classify violent behavior more homogenously. In children with CD, it has been shown that ADHD is a moderator of reactive but not proactive aggression [38]. Bennett et al. [39] demonstrated in 8- to 15-year-old children that reactive antisocial behavior is more related to ADHD than proactive antisocial behavior.

Following the hypothesis that reactive violence and not proactive violence might be related to ADHD, we performed an exploratory study with 66 males who had committed different types of violent offences. We found a strong association between the presence of ADHD and reactive violence (OR 2.7, 95% CI 1.5– 107.9) [40]. In contrast, proactive violence was more prominent in offenders without ADHD. These findings appear plausible as reactive violence is not planned but always spontaneous, a reaction to a provocation or a conflict and is driven by affective outbursts. It is short-lived and has no finalistic target except the reduction of tension and agitation. Usually, reactive violence is not rational but impulsive and there is no systematic or instrumental character of the criminal action. Thus, according to these criteria, reactive violence has significant overlap in character with the psychopathology of ADHD.

ADHD-Associated Antisociality and APD without ADHD

During the past decade there was a vivid discussion concerning the role of ADHD in terms of adult criminality and APD. From a genetic perspective it has been argued that ADHD and comorbid CD might be a more severe variant of ADHD and not distinct disorders [41–43]. According to the epidemiologic studies and follow-up research there is overwhelming evidence that about one-half of the ADHD children seem to develop later CD (see fig. 1). From this subsample another half displays the symptoms of APD during adulthood [9, 27, 28, 44]. Indeed, ADHD+APD is a common diagnosis in forensic psychiatry. Referring to a worldwide prevalence of 0.034 of ADHD in adults [1] and a prevalence of up to 0.03 of APD [45], the co-occurrence of ADHD and APD can be calculated as 0.001, if both disorders occur independently. However, as mentioned above, in forensic psychiatric populations the observed prevalence of ADHD+APD is at least 100 times higher.

The nature of the association between the two disorders is not fully understood so far. Genetic factors contribute substantially to the risk of developing both conditions, although specific genes that affect the development of APD in ADHD have yet to be identified [41, 46]. ADHD severity of psychopathology and the disease pervasiveness might be predictors of antisocial behavior [46]. Antisocial behavior is also linked with familial adversity as well as peer rejection. Disrupted parental discipline might also be a common factor to increase the risk for APD in ADHD [47]. According to the results of the prospective follow-up study by Satterfield et al. [22, 23], low socio-economic status and IQ were unspecific risk factors that could predict a higher prevalence of antisocial activities in ADHD individuals.

It has already been mentioned that adult APD and criminality in children with ADHD can be best predicted by comorbid CD. The item content of CD gives a hint why it is possible to predict later antisociality and criminal behavior by childhood-onset or adolescent-onset CD (table 2).

Table 2. DSM-IV definition of CD. 11 items are accentuated with x. These definitions correspond directly to definitions of the penal law. For a diagnosis of CD, 3 symptoms during 1 year must be present

Diagnostic criteria of DSM-IV for CD	
Aggression towards people and animals	
1. Threatens, bullies or intimidates others	x
2. Often initiates physical fights	x
3. Has used a weapon that can cause severe harm	x
4. Physically cruel to people	x
5. Physically cruel to animals	x
6. Has stolen while confronting a victim	x
7. Has forced someone into sexual activity	x
Destruction of property	
8. Has deliberately engaged in fire-setting	x
9. Has deliberately destroyed others' property	x
Deceitfulness or theft	
10. Has broken into someone else's house, car, etc.	x
11. Often lies to obtain goods or to avoid obligations	
12. Has stolen items of non-trivial value (shoplifting)	x
Serious violations of rules	
13. Often stays out at night before the age 13 years	
14. Has run away from home overnight while living in a surrogate home	
15. Is often truant from school, beginning before the age 13 years	

The diagnostic criteria of CD point directly to the paragraphs of the criminal code. Out of 15 items, 11 refer to definitions of the penal law. The remaining 4 items (11, 13, 14, 15) are not psychopathologic in nature but clearly indicate severe rule-breaking behaviors. Facing the list of behaviors from table 2, a judge or a criminologist would say this is apparently childhood or adolescent delinquency. The diagnostic concept of APD follows similar rules. Of 7 diagnostic criteria, 4 refer fully or partly to criminal behavior. Only 3 of 7 criteria must be fulfilled to make the diagnosis. Thus it is apparent that persons with different and recidivistic crimes have a high risk of getting the APD diagnosis. The overlap of symptoms of CD, ASP and criminality is massive and explains why CD is a potent predictor of later antisociality or criminality. This is in accordance with widely accepted results of criminologic research. The best predictor for future crime is earlier crime [48]. This conclusion, however, does not help to elucidate the link between ADHD and APD. So far, beside the above-mentioned genetic and environmental hypotheses, little is known about what risk factors and mechanisms contribute to the frequent association of ADHD and APD.

In the given frame it is interesting to investigate whether the antisociality associated with ADHD differs from antisociality in persons without ADHD. The concept of psychopathy [49], which has found general acceptance in forensic psychiatry, refers to a core population of antisocial individuals. This is a construct dating to the beginning of the 19th century when Prichard [50] described the psychopathology of moral insanity. The psychopathology of psychopathy refers to symptoms like shallow affect, superficial charm, manipulativeness, lack of empathy, etc. Psychopathy is associated with poor treatment response and the forensic prognosis is in almost all cases unfavorable. The psychopathology of the psychopaths can be assessed by the Psychopathy Checklist (PCL-R) [51]. Scores derived from this scale are valid risk factors indicating criminal offences and in particular violent behavior. Thus the PCL-R is part of the most widely accepted risk assessment procedures for violent or sexual offences like the HCR-20 [52] and the SVR-20 [53]. Psychopaths are a small population, but they account for an excess of felony crimes and for criminal recidivism. An association between ADHD and the psychopathy concept could be assumed since there is certain overlap between the DSM-IV items referring to the ADHD syndrome impulsivity and the PCL factor focusing on poor behavior control and impulsivity. Thus we conducted a study with 230 incarcerated men. All had committed felony crimes and were incarcerated for more than 2 years. The screening version of the PCL was administered for the assessment of psychopathy. ADHD syndrome scores were established by means of the ADHD self-report scale [54, 55]. The instrument consists of the 18 DSM-IV criteria that can be graduated from 0 until 3 on a Lickert Scale. We found a rank correlation of 0.2 between the PCL-SV and the ADHD-SR, which was statistically significant ($p \leq 0.01$). Despite the statistical significance it is obvious that a correlation of 0.2 cannot make a claim for clinical meaningfulness.

In order to investigate further the possible associations between the psychopathy items and the criteria of ADHD, we performed a factor analysis. Our expectation was that in the case of an association between ADHD and psychopathy, common factors of psychopathology should be present (table 3).

The solution with seven factors accounted for 60% of the variance. No factor was found consisting of items from both concepts. There were 3 pure ADHD and 4 pure psychopathy factors. It is apparent that there was no association between diagnostic items of ADHD with those of psychopathy. Thus both psychopathological concepts seemed to be unrelated. In view of these results there might be a difference between psychopathic antisociality and antisociality with ADHD with regard to the course of the disorder. At present, psychopathic antisociality is thought to be a robust disorder with a lifelong perspective which is indicative for the worst forensic prognosis. In contrast, ADHD-associated antisociality may be limited to the second and third decades of life. Our results are in line with findings reported just recently by Fowler et al. [56], who found single psychopathic traits in adolescents with ADHD but the PCL scores were below the range of typical psychopathy.

Table 3. Factor analysis including 18 ADHD items (DSM-IV) and 12 psychopathy criteria (PCL-SV). 7 factors were extracted in accordance to the classical eigenvalue (>1) criterion. No overlap between ADHD and psychopathy items could be detected

	Factor analysis ADHD and psychopathy items						
	F1	F2	F3	F4	F5	F6	F7
ADHD							
1. Careless mistakes	0.45	0.44					
2. Sustaining attention	0.65						
3. Does not listen when spoken to		0.46					
4. Does not follow instructions		0.57					
5. Organizing tasks		0.61					
6. Avoids mental efforts		0.52					
7. Loses things		0.59					
8. External stimuli		0.70					
9. Forgetful		0.72					
10. Fidgets/squirms	0.81						
11. Leaves seat	0.76						
12. Restlessness	0.77						
13. Not quiet	0.44	0.39	0.35				
14. Driven by a motor	0.42		0.45				
15. Talks excessively			0.79				
16. Blurts out	0.37		0.46				
17. Difficulty waiting		0.61					
18. Interrupts others			0.72				
Psychopathy (PCL-SV)							
1. Superficial						0.67	
2. Grandiosity						0.70	
3. Manipulative						0.58	
4. Lack of remorse					0.75		
5. Lack of empathy					0.61		
6. Responsibility					0.76		
7. Impulsivity				0.76			
8. Poor behavioral control				0.78			
9. No long-term goals				0.67			
10. Irresponsibility				0.51	0.49		
11. Juvenile antisociality				0.53			0.58
12. Adult antisociality							0.80

Conclusion

There are several lines of evidence allowing for a more precise conceptualization in which way ADHD could play a role in the development of antisocial and criminal behavior. The main aspect is that the risk to develop later antisociality or criminality is mediated by comorbid CD and not by ADHD itself. ADHD with early-onset CD can be differentiated from ADHD with adolescent-onset CD. About 50% of the individuals with ADHD and CD develop later ASP. The prevalence of ADHD associated with CD or ASP in offender populations is increased. The highest prevalences were detected in male adolescents and young male adults. In principle, the situation in female offenders and forensic populations is similar, but the prevalence of ADHD with CD or APD does not seem to be as high when compared with men. In both genders the prevalence decreases remarkably with advancing age. This supports the notion that ADHD in combination with antisociality may not play a significant role in individuals with life-course persistent antisociality.

When comparing offender populations with and without ADHD it becomes apparent that ADHD has a modulating effect on the onset and the risk for recidivistic offending. ADHD has apparently not much to do with those offences which have an instrumental, systematic and finalistic character, and which are deliberate and planned with foresight. A characteristic example is fraud where the prevalence of ADHD is in a normal range. ADHD plays a significant role in sexual delinquency and reactive violent offences, whereas in proactive violence ADHD has a low prevalence.

APD is one of the most frequent comorbid conditions in ADHD. The coincidence of ADHD and APD in offender populations is at least 100 times higher if it would be left to chance. Contrary to earlier expectations, the forensic or criminal outcome of persons with ADHD/CD/APD might not necessarily be unfavorable. There is growing evidence that persons with these conditions have a remarkable remission rate during the third and fourth decades of their lives. Moreover, males with ADHD do not belong to the core group of psychopaths [51] who are markedly overrepresented in all sorts of delinquency including severe felony crime and recidivistic crime.

Beside CD, oppositional defiant disorder is a further comorbid condition of ADHD beginning during childhood. The effects of CD and oppositional defiant disorder on the course of ADHD are discussed by R. Klein in this volume.

References

1 Fayyad J, De Graf R, Kessler R, Alonso J, Angermeyer M, Demyttenaere K, De Girolamo G, Haro M, Karam EG, Lara C, Lepine JP, Ormel J, Posada-Villa J, Zaslavsky AM, Jin T: Cross-national prevalence and correlates of adult attention-deficit hyperactivity disorder. Br J Psychiatry 2007;190:402–409.

2 Kessler RC, Adler L, Barkley R, Biederman J, Conners CK, Demler O, Faraone S, Greenhill LL, Howes MJ, Secnik K, Spencer T, Ustun TB, Walters EE, Zaslavsky AM: The prevalence and correlates of adult ADHD in the United States: results from the National Comorbidity Survey Replication. Am J Psychiatry 2006;163:716–723.

3 Wender PH: Attention-Deficit Hyperactivity Disorder in Adults. New York, Oxford University Press, 1995.

4 Reimherr FW, Marchant BK, Strong RE, Hedges DW, Adler L, Spencer TJ, West SA, Soni P: Emotional dysregulation in adult ADHD and response to atomoxetine. Biol Psychiatry 2005;58:125–131.

5 Reimherr FW, Williams ED, Strong RE, Mestas R, Soni P, Marchant BK: A double-blind, placebo-controlled, crossover study of osmotic release oral system methylphenidate in adults with ADHD with assessment of oppositional and emotional dimensions of the disorder. J Clin Psychiatry 2007;68:93–101.

6 Conners CK, Erhardt D, Sparrow E: CAARS – Adult ADHD Rating Scales: Technical Manual. New York, MHS, 1999.
7 Rösler M, Retz W, Retz-Junginger P, Stieglitz RD, Kessler H, Reimherr F, Wender PH: Attention deficit hyperactivity disorder in adults. Benchmarking diagnosis using the Wender-Reimherr Adult ADHD Rating Scale (in German). Nervenarzt 2008;79:320–327.
8 Barkley RA: Major life activity and health outcomes associated with attention-deficit/hyperactivity disorder. J Clin Psychiatry 2002;63(suppl 12):10–15.
9 Weiss G, Hechtman LT, Milroy T, Perlman T: Psychiatric status of hyperactives as adults: a controlled prospective 15-year follow-up of 63 hyperactive children. J Am Acad Child Psychiatry 1985;24:211–220.
10 Mannuzza S, Klein RG, Bessler A, Malloy P, LaPadula M: Adult outcome of hyperactive boys: educational achievement, occupational rank, and psychiatric status. Arch Gen Psychiatry 1993;50:565–576.
11 Mannuzza S, Klein RG, Bessler A, Malloy P, Lapadula M: Adult psychiatric status of hyperactive boys grown up. Am J Psychiatry 1998;155:493–498.
12 Barkley RA, Fischer M., Smallish L, Fletcher K: Young adult outcome of hyperactive children; adaptive functioning in major life activities. J Am Acad Child Adolesc Psychiatry 2006;45:192–202.
13 Grützmacher H: Unfallgefährdung bei Aufmerksamkeits- und Hyperaktivitätsstörung. Dtsch Ärzteblatt 2001;98:1898–190.
14 Kaya A, Taner Y, Guclu B, Taner E, Kaya Y, Bahcivan HG, Benli IT: Trauma and adult attention deficit hyperactivity disorder. J Int Med Res 2008;36:9–16.
15 Jerome L, Habinski L, Segal A: Attention-deficit/hyperactivity disorder and driving risk: a review of the literature and a methodological critique. Curr Psychiatry Rep 2006;8:416–426.
16 Vermeiren R: Psychopathology and delinquency in adolescents: a descriptive and developmental perspective. Clin Psychol Rev 2003;23:277–318.
17 Timmons-Mitchel J, Brown C, Schulz SC, Webster SE, Underwood LA, Semple WE: Comparing the mental health needs of female and male incarcerated juvenile delinquents. Behav Sci Law 1997;15:195–202.
18 Ulzen T, Hamilton H: The nature and characteristics of psychiatric comorbidity in incarcerated adolescents. Can J Psychiatry 1998;43:57–63.
19 Rösler M, Retz W, Retz-Junginger P, Hengesch G, Schneider M, Supprian T, Schwitzgebel P, Pinhard K, Dovi-Akue N, Wender P, Thome J: Prevalence of attention-deficit hyperactivity disorder in male young adult prison inmates. Eur Arch Psychiatry Clin Neurosci 2004;254:365–371.
20 Babinski LM, Hartsough CS, Lambert NM: Childhood conduct problems, hyperactivity-impulsivity, and inattention as predictors of adult criminal activity. J Child Psychol Psychiatry 1999;40:347–355.
21 Loeber R, Green SM, Keenan K, Lahey BB: Which boys will fare worse? Early predictors of the onset of conduct disorder in a six-year longitudinal study. J Am Acad Child Adolesc Psychiatry 1995;34:499–509.
22 Satterfield J, Hoppe C, Schell A: A prospective study of delinquency in 110 adolescent boys with attention deficit disorder and 88 normal adolescent boys. Am J Psychiatry 1982;139:795–798.
23 Satterfield JH, Faller KJ, Crinella FM, Schell AM, Swansson JM, Homer LD: A 30-year prospective follow-up study of hyperactive boys with conduct problems: adult criminality. J Am Acad Child Adolesc Psychiatry 2007;46:601–610.
24 Lahey BB, Loeber R, Burke JD, Applegate B: Predicting future antisocial personality disorder in males from a clinical assessment in childhood. J Consult Clin Psychology 2005;73:389–399.
25 Taylor E, Chadwick O, Heptinstall E, Dankaerts M: Hyperactivity and conduct problems as risk factors for adolescent development. J Am Acad Child Adolesc Psychiatry 1996;35:1213–1226.
26 Gunter TD, Arndt S, Riggins-Capder K, Wenman G, Cadoret RJ: Adult outcomes of attention deficit hyperactivity disorder and conduct disorder: are the risks independent or additive? Ann Clin Psychiatry 2006;18:223–237.
27 Satterfield JH, Schell A: A prospective study of hyperactive boys with conduct problems and normal boys: adolescent and adult criminality. J Child Adolesc Psychiatry 1997;36:1726–1735.
28 Barkley RA, Fischer M, Smallish L, Fletcher K: Young adult follow-up of hyperactive children: antisocial activities and drug use. J Child Psychol Psychiatry 2004;45:195–211.
29 Mannuzza S, Klein RG, Moulton JL: Lifetime criminality among boys with attention deficit hyperactivity disorder: a prospective follow-up study into adulthood using official arrest records. Psychiatry Res 2008;160:237–246.
30 Moffitt TE: Life-course-persistent and adolescent-limited antisocial behavior: a 10-year research review and research agenda; in Lahey BB, Moffitt TE, Capdi A (eds): Causes of conduct disorder and juvenile delinquency. New York, Guilford Press, 2003.
31 Rösler M, Retz W, Yaqoobi K, Burg E, Retz-Junginger P: Attention deficit/hyperactivity disorder in female offenders: prevalence, psychiatric comorbidity and psychosocial implications. Eur Arch Psychiatry Clin Neurosci 2009;258:98–105.

32 Moffitt TE: Juvenile delinquency and attention deficit disorder: boys' developmental trajectories from age 3 to age 15. Child Dev 1990:61:893–910.
33 Ziegler E, Blocher D, Gross J, Rösler M: Assessment of attention-deficit hyperactivity disorder in prison inmates. Recht Psychiatrie 2003;21:17–21.
34 Blocher D, Henkel K, Retz W, Retz-Junginger P, Thome J, Rösler M: Symptome aus dem Spektrum des hyperkinetischen Syndroms bei Sexualdelinquenten. Fortschr Neurol Psychiatr 2001;69:453–459.
35 Rösler M: ADHD is linked to reactive violent and antisocial behaviour but not to psychopathy. J Neural Transm 2007;114:LII.
36 Dodge KA, Coie JD: Social information processing factors in reactive and proactive aggression in children's peer groups. J Pers Soc Psychol 1987;53:1146–1158.
37 Vitiello B, Stoff DM: Subtypes of aggression and their relevance to child psychiatry. J Am Acad Child Adolesc Psychiatry 1997;23:277–318.
38 Waschbusch DA, Wiloughby MT: Attention-deficit/hyperactivity disorder and callous-unemotional traits as moderators of conduct problems when examining impairment and aggression in elementary school children. Aggress Behav 2007;33:1–15.
39 Bennett DS, Pitale M, Vora V, Rheingold AA: Reactive vs. proactive antisocial behavior: differential correlates of child ADHD symptoms? J Atten Dis 2004;7:197–204.
40 Retz W, Rösler M: Gewalttätiges Verhalten bei Straftätern mit ADHS: Assoziation mit reaktiver aber nicht mit proaktiver Gewalt. Nervenarzt 2007; 78(suppl 2):206.
41 Thapar A, Harrington R, McGuffin P: Examining the comorbidity of ADHD-related behaviours and conduct problems using a twin study design. Br J Psychiatry 2001;179:224–229.
42 Nadder TS, Rutter M, Silberg JL, Maes HH, Eaves LJ: Genetic effects on the variation and covariation of attention deficit-hyperactivity disorder and oppositional-defiant disorder/conduct disorder symptomatologies across informant and occasion of measurement. Psychol Med 2002;32:39–53.
43 Dick DM, Viken RJ, Kaprio J, Pulkkinen L, Rose RJ: Understanding the covariation among childhood externalizing symptoms: genetic and environmental influences on conduct disorder, attention deficit hyperactivity disorder, and oppositional defiant disorder symptoms. J Abnorm Child Psychol 2005;33: 219–229.
44 Mannuzza S, Klein RG, Konig PH, Giampino TL: Hyperactive boys almost grown up. IV. Criminality and its relationship to psychiatric status. Arch Gen Psychiatry 1989;46:1073–1079.
45 Moran P: The epidemiology of antisocial personality disorder. Soc Psychiatry Psychiatr Epidemiol 1999;34:231–242.
46 Thapar A, van den Bree M, Fowler T, Langley K, Whittinger N: Predictors of antisocial behaviour in children with attention deficit hyperactivity disorder. Eur Child Adolesc Psychiatry 2006;15:118–125.
47 Patterson GR, DeGarmo DS, Knutson N: Hyperactive and antisocial behaviours: comorbid or two points of the same process? Dev Psychopathol 2002;12:91–106.
48 Monahan J, Steadman HJ, Appelbaum PS, Robbins PC, Mulvey EP, Silver E, Roth LH, Grisso T: Developing a clinically useful actuarial tool for assessing violence risk. Br J Psychiatry 2000;176:312–319.
49 Hare RD: Psychopathy: a clinical construct whose time has come. Crim Justice Behav 1996;23:25–54.
50 Prichard JC: The Treatise of Insanity and Other Disorders Affecting the Mind. London, Sherwood, Gilbert & Piper, 1835.
51 Hare RD, Harpur TJ, Hakstian AR, Forth AE, Hart SD, Newman JP: The revised psychopathy checklist: descriptive statistics, reliability, and factor structure. Psychological assessment. J Consult Clin Psychol 1990;2:228–341.
52 Webster CD, Douglas KS, Eaves D, Hart SD: Assessing Risk for Violence Version 2. Mental Health, Law and Policy Institute. Burnaby, Simon Frazer University, 1997.
53 Boer DP, Hart SD, Kropp PR, Webster CD: Sexual violence risk-20 (SVR-20). Mental Health, Law, and Policy Institute. Burnaby, Simon Fraser University, 1997.
54 Rösler M, Retz W, Thome J, Schneider M, Stieglitz R-D, Falkai P: Psychopathological rating scales for diagnostic use in adults with attention deficit/hyperactivity disorder Eur Arch Psychiatry Clin Neurosci 2006;256(suppl 1):3–11.
55 Rösler M, Retz-Junginger P, Retz W, Stieglitz R-D: Homburger ADHS-Skalen für Erwachsene (HASE). Göttingen, Hogrefe, 2008.
56 Fowler T, Lanley K, Rice F, Whittinger N, Ross K, van Goozen S, Owen MJ, O'Donovan MC, van den Bree, Thapar A: Psychopathy traits in adolescents with childhood attention-deficit hyperactivity disorder. Br J Psychiatry 2009;194:62–67.
57 Hollander HE, Turner FD: Characteristics of incarcerated delinquents: relationship between developmental disorders, environmental and family factors, and patterns of offence and recidivism. J Am Acad Child Adolesc Psychiatry 1985;24:221–226.
58 Milin R, Halikas JA, Meller JE, Morse C: Psychopathology among substance abusing juvenile offenders. J Am Acad Child Adolesc Psychiatry 1991; 30:569–574.

59 Haapasalo J, Hämäläinen T: Childhood family problems and current psychiatric problems among young violent and property offenders. J Am Acad Child Adolesc Psychiatry 1996;35:1394–1401.
60 Richards J: Psychiatric disorders among adolescents in custody. Aust NZ J Psychiatry 1996;30:788–793.
61 Doreleijers TAH, Moser F, This P, van Engeland H, Beyaert FHL: Forensic assessment of juvenile delinquents: prevalence of psychopathology and decision-making at court in The Netherlands. J Adolescence 2000;23:263–275.
62 Pliszka SR, Sherman JO, Barrow WV, Irick S: Affective disorders in juvenile offenders: a preliminary study. Am J Psychiatry 2000;157:130–132.
63 Vermeiren R, De Clippele A, Deboutte D: A descriptive survey of Flemish adolescent delinquents. J Adolesc 2000;23:277–285.
64 Ruchkin V, Koposov R, Vermeiren R, Schwab-Stone M: Psychopathology and age of onset of conduct problems in juvenile delinquents. J Clin Psychiatry 2003;64:913–920.
65 Retz W, Rösler M: The relation of ADHD and violent aggression: What can we learn from epidemiological and genetic studies? Int J Law Psychiatry 2009; May, epub ahead of print.

Prof. Michael Rösler, MD
Neurocentre, Saarland University Hospital
Institute for Forensic Psychology and Psychiatry
DE–66421 Homburg/Saar (Germany)
Tel. +49 0 6841 1626350, Fax +49 0 6841 1626335, E-Mail michael.roesler@uks.eu

Retz W, Klein RG (eds): Attention-Deficit Hyperactivity Disorder (ADHD) in Adults.
Key Issues in Mental Health. Basel, Karger, 2010, vol 176, pp 159–173

Psychotherapy in Adult Attention-Deficit Hyperactivity Disorder

Alexandra Philipsen · Harald Richter · Swantje Matthies · Bernd Hesslinger

Department of Psychiatry and Psychotherapy, University of Freiburg Medical School, Freiburg, Germany

Abstract

In contrast to the treatment of attention-deficit hyperactivity disorder (ADHD) in children and adolescents, few disorder-oriented psychotherapeutic approaches are currently available for the treatment of adults with ADHD. The development and the empirical examination of these began chiefly in the last years. Prior to 2002, various clinical interventions were described and emphasis was placed on different problem areas in the literature, but no empirical data on the effectiveness of different concepts was available. On the whole, suggestions for treatment concerned psychoeducation for ADHD as a chronic disorder, help with the structuring of daily life, self-organization, interventions in the interpersonal domain, and problems of self-esteem. The first therapy studies were published in 2002 in which structured treatment programs were evaluated. This article provides an overview of the treatment approaches and of selected empirical studies on the effectiveness of psychotherapy in adults with ADHD. Following this, a validated and manualized treatment concept will be described as an exemplary approach. Finally, the specific requirements of psychotherapy for ADHD in adults and on further research will be discussed.

In contrast to the treatment of attention-deficit hyperactivity disorder (ADHD) in children and adolescents there are currently few disorder-oriented options for the psychotherapeutic treatment of adults. The development and empirical examination of these treatments only just began in the last years. A chief reason for this is that the disorder in adults has only received the greater attention of the scientific and therapeutic community in more recent years. In view of the pronounced biological nature of this disorder, the initial approach to the therapeutic intervention was to place the emphasis on medication for which clear-cut proof of its effectiveness in children and adolescents had already been delivered.

Although medication has played a crucial part in improving the core symptoms of ADHD of many patients and has therefore become established as a keystone of therapy, the clinical experience in the treatment of adult patients demonstrates that medication alone is often insufficient in meeting the needs of adult patients for whom secondary psychosocial consequences and comorbid disorders, rather than the core symptoms, are of prime importance in adult age. Further to this, many patients do not want treatment based on medication alone. They prefer either supplementary psychotherapeutic treatment or, because of concerns about stimulants, treatment on a psychotherapeutic basis only.

The biography of many patients is dotted with psychotherapeutic treatments which were entered into following most diverse diagnoses, treatments that were very often discontinued because the patients labored under the impression that their specific needs were not being given sufficient consideration.

Specific Approaches to Treatment

There are reviews in the psychotherapeutic literature for disorder-oriented treatment that describe several clinical interventions and spotlight different problem areas. Empirical data on the effectiveness of different concepts were however not available until 2002 [1–6]. The main elements of proposed treatments included psychoeducation for ADHD as a chronic disorder, help and support in structuring daily life, acquisition of skills in planning, and self-organization. Recommendations were made for coping with the interpersonal ramifications of the disorder. These included counseling of family members and spouses, training of social skills, and participation in self-help groups. As further important elements, interventions for the improvement of self-esteem as well as general 'coaching' entered into therapy proposals.

In these programs, treatment instructions for therapists mostly include suggestions for a generally supportive and encouraging mindset and attitude toward patients. Some programs recommended a medication and psychotherapy-based combination therapy or a graduated approach in which the core symptoms are treated first with medication and residual problems subsequently treated psychotherapeutically [4]. While the programs for structuring of daily routine and for imparting skills rested largely on behavioral-therapeutic principles, depth-psychological approaches focused particularly on the problems of self-esteem [7, 8]. Considerations and reports of the positive influence of group settings on conducting therapy were already considered and reported within the framework of these therapy recommendations [e.g. 9].

Previous Psychotherapy Studies

Disorder-Oriented Group Programs

Two papers were published in 2002 [10, 11] that reported the positive effect of a structured disorder-oriented behavioral therapy on adult patients with ADHD. In this study by an Australian study group, a standardized group program was carried out that comprised 8 weekly, 2-hour sessions and provided support for participants through coaching by students and through homework based on the treatment material. The aim was to improve the patients' ability to self-organize, control anger, reduce impulse control, and to improve self-esteem. The investigated groups comprised 22 patients and a control group of 21 patients with and without medication. Medication was maintained at a stable level throughout the period of the investigation. The results showed a reduction in the ADHD symptoms and an improvement in self-esteem and organization. The 1-year follow-up confirmed stable improvements.

The study by our work group [10] investigated 8 patients, initially within the context of a controlled clinical trial, with a group program made up of 13 weekly group sessions and optional individual sessions. The control group comprised 7 waiting-list patients. Medication, where administered, was stable throughout. The data from the measured self-report scales (ADHD symptoms, depression, general psychopathology, and well-being) showed significant improvements in the treatment group in the pre/post comparison. Patient satisfaction with the therapy was also measured and proved to be very high. A subsequent open multicenter feasibility study at four university sites with a total of 72 patients was largely able to replicate these results and proving therapist- and group-independent effectiveness [12]. Only 8% did not complete the treatment. Patients rated the topics mindfulness, behavioral analysis and emotion regulation as most effective for their improvement and the group setting and the support of the therapists were regarded as equally helpful (see below for the principles and content of this group treatment program). These findings go along with a recent feasibility study on a mindfulness training program based on the stress reduction concept of Jon Kabat-Zinn with eight sessions lasting 2.5 h each and daily at-home practice (for maximally 15 min). 25 of 32 adults and adolescents completed the study. Mindfulness training resulted in significant pre- to post-treatment improvements with regard to ADHD and associated symptoms (depression, anxiety, impulsivity) [13]. Moreover, there were neurocognitive benefits reported, particularly concerning attention conflict and set shifting.

Disorder-Oriented Individual Programs

A pilot study [14] was published in 2004 on the implementation of the cognitive behavioral therapy according to Beck in single therapy settings for ADHD patients. In this study by McDermott et al., 26 patients were treated for over 1 year in single sessions. On average, 36 sessions per patient were performed. 85% of the patients were on medication. The content of the therapy incorporated various cognitive interventions for recognition and restructuring of negative thoughts as well as for learning techniques of problem-solving and for organization skills. The variables ADHD, anxiety, depression, and general level of functioning were investigated. Clear improvements in 69% of the patients were reported. The authors see some indication of the effectiveness of their procedure, but interpret their results with some caution on account of the absence of a control group and insufficient control of the pharmacological treatment. A further controlled study on cognitive behavioral therapy was published in 2005 by the work group around Safren et al. [15]. Patients presenting clear symptoms following a medication-based therapy underwent additional psychotherapeutic treatment. The patients were randomly assigned to the conditions 'medication-based therapy vs. non-medication-based therapy' and 'cognitive behavioral therapy'. 31 patients were investigated, psychotherapy encompassed 11 settings. The content comprised modules on organization, coping with distraction, and cognitive interventions for dysfunctional thoughts. Further themes were, if needed, communication training and coping with anger. Significant improvements were found in the variables ADHD symptoms, anxiety, depression, and general well-being. The response rate differentiated significantly between the two groups (56% combined treatment, 13% medication only). These results substantiate the hypotheses on the effectiveness of psychotherapy for residual symptoms after pharmacotherapy.

A further study on cognitive behavioral therapy in which the therapeutic procedure was however not manualized is reported by Rostain and Ramsay [16]. 43 ADHD-investigated patients underwent a 5-month cognitive behavioral therapy and were administered amphetamines. As all patients of the study received amphetamines commitment to behavioral therapy, and because the majority of them had a current comorbid anxiety or depression disorder, a conclusive assessment of the specific contribution of the psychotherapy to the described improvements was not possible.

Weiss and Hechtman [17] published a study that dealt not only with the psychological impact of ADHD but also with the functional impairments associated with ADHD. Their criticism of the other described studies concerns the failure of these to investigate the functional impairments. In a therapy that took a problem-oriented behavioral therapeutic approach to the ADHD problematic and administered stimulants, Weiss and Hechtman investigated a group of 96 patients over a period of 5 months. This study demonstrated a correlation between the improvement in psychosocial impairments and the improvement in functional symptoms.

Adaptation of Individual Programs for Group Settings

Interestingly, the cognitive behavioral therapy program has been also adapted for a group setting with 3 monthly 1-day workshops over a period of 6 months and evaluated in a controlled study with 61 adult ADHD patients (medication vs. combination treatment [18]). The combination therapy led to significant improvements of knowledge of ADHD, self-esteem and self-efficacy compared to the control group. The group setting was regarded as highly effective for their improvements by the patients. Depression and anxiety was equally reduced in both groups.

Classification of the Psychotherapeutic Concepts to Date and the Requirements Placed on a Disorder-Oriented Psychotherapy

The studies to date appear to speak in favor of the effectiveness of psychotherapeutic interventions for adults with ADHD, even though there are still numerous issues to be resolved and despite the necessity for further empirical research. On the basis of the presented concepts and the growing clinical experience in the application of programs, a number of different conclusions may be drawn and requirements of psychotherapeutic treatments of ADHD in adults formulated.

In order that the special features of the disorder with its different cognitive, affective and psychosocial impairments are taken into account, the treatment programs need to give the following points their due consideration:

- Clarification and psychoeducation should form a substantial part of the treatment [19]. Although many adults with ADHD are relieved to receive an explanatory model of the different aspects of their problems, dealing with this new information can be all the more difficult for them. Many of those affected have already experienced years or even decades of adapting to the problems prior to receiving a diagnosis. In contrast to other mental problems that emerge in the course of adulthood, these patients have experienced themselves as being different since their childhood and have in part internalized the attributions of their environment about the causal conditions of their particular characteristics in their self-image, or they find themselves in a permanent state of contention with their environment ('Have I got a problem or has everyone else got a problem with me?'). The fundamental destabilization of the self-concept that results from this is an important factor that needs to be considered.
- The emotional instability and its impact on relationships and on social functioning can come to the fore in adulthood and should be given due consideration.
- For those affected, the symptoms of ADHD do not only present problems in their social environment but are also potential disruptive factors for the execution of the psychotherapy that need therefore to be considered. Disorder-typical behavior can be expected that will frustrate the therapeutic setting (forgetting appointments, unpunctuality, difficulties in managing homework, etc.). These disrupting influences on the therapy need to be born in mind both prior to and during the course of the therapy when choosing the setting and when preparing and arranging the therapy.
- The frequent occurrence of comorbid disorders means that the psychotherapy should have suggestions for a hierarchical approach for dealing with these comorbidities and should consider the particular consequences of this.
- Not all manifestations of ADHD require treatment in adulthood. There are nevertheless many affected who hope for improvement in the quality of life, even though they have already achieved a very high level of functioning in other areas ('high functioning ADHD'). There is therefore a fluid transition to coaching and

'personal growth' approaches. A psychotherapeutic concept that takes this into account should be constructed in a modular fashion in order to enable the patient and the therapist to target individual problem areas, according to individual assessment.
- Given that the symptoms of ADHD in adulthood are interindividually very different and that for many the aim is to control the disorder and not to 'eliminate' it, the notion of improving the self-management of the debilitating effects of the disease should be given priority. Many of those affected report that they do not wish to see their lives without certain facets of ADHD.

The Freiburg Treatment Program as an Example of a Disorder-Oriented Therapy Concept with Several Therapy Modules

A treatment program, in development since 1999 at the University Clinic Freiburg, will be presented in the following in greater detail as an example of a standardized and evaluated disorder-oriented treatment program [10, 12, 20]. It is presented also because this procedure is currently further investigated in a larger randomized study [21].

The main objective in developing this disorder-oriented group program was to improve the control of (but not 'heal') the symptoms of ADHD ('To control ADHD rather than being controlled by ADHD').

Further aims were:
- Experience of enhanced control, based on information in the form of a disorder-specific psychoeducation;
- Positive influence on the core symptoms (attentional disorders, hyperactivity, impulse control, disorganization and affect disorders) through specific training of skills;
- Improved coping with the psychosocial consequences of the symptomatic (work, relationships);
- Improvement of the mostly low or instable self-esteem, and
- Achieve a balance between 'accepting' the symptoms and 'altering' them in the sense of an active and responsible coping approach to their consequences.

Basic Principles

The starting point for the development of a therapy concept was the transfer of the general therapeutic factors of psychotherapy according to Grawe [22] and the concept of dialectic behavioral therapy of borderline personality disorder according to Linehan [23]. The transfer of the concept has to consider the following points:

Clarification

The therapy should create a frame of reference in which those aspects of experience and behavior that encroach upon the patient meeting his or her basic needs, and therefore upon the patient's life quality, can be described as treatable symptoms of ADHD. Information about the causes, symptoms, diagnostics and treatment possibilities are therefore central elements of the treatment: 'What do I have, why, what do I want to change, how do I go about it?'

Resource Activation

Imparting a balanced view of ADHD is of focal importance in a resource-oriented approach: 'ADHD imposes limitations – but it presents many possibilities (e.g., creativity, prepared to take risks, fantasy), too. How can you use your resources in order to set about achieving the goals defined in the clarification phase?'

The induction of positive change expectancies is held to be a specific therapeutic factor in hypnotherapy procedures. A central element of therapeutic approaches should be the induction of expectancies of improvement that in a secondary fashion can evoke positive feedback processes [22].

Problem Actualization

Many individuals with ADHD experience difficulties with the concrete analysis of problematic behavior. Even before it comes to a detailed behavioral analysis, acquired behavioral patterns frequently cause the patient to jump to a level of explanation or justification that is frequently connected with a rapid change of self- and other attributions about the root cause ('Who is to blame'?). In order to accomplish problem actuation it would therefore appear sensible to firstly recognize the problem behavior as ADHD-typical behavior in order to then develop coping strategies, to exercise these in concrete situations, and to subsequently transfer these to comparable situations ('exercise, exercise, exercise').

Coping

The described transfer leads to a long-term generalization of both problem-solving at the behavioral level and of change in attribution patterns in the sense of a more stable self- and other perception and a change in the self-image and experienced control.

The Dialectic Behavioral Therapy of Borderline Personality Disorder, developed by Linehan [23] at the University of Washington in Seattle, USA, is an empirically investigated therapy model that is very similar to this one in the symptoms it focuses on, in the considerations paid to structuring the therapeutic settings and in its described objectives.

From a phenomenological point of view there are some similarities between ADHD and borderline personality disorder: deficits in affect regulation, impulse control, substance abuse, low self-esteem and disturbed interpersonal relationship are common in both conditions [24–26]. In ADHD, attention deficit is most pronounced in situations which lack external stimulation. In contrast, patients with borderline personality disorder often experience dissociative symptoms when they feel emotionally stressed. From a neurophysiological point of view, dissociation in borderline personality disorder might be regarded as a special form of attention deficit [24].

Mechanisms of affect regulation, however, differ quite dramatically in the two conditions. Patients with ADHD, the majority being male, often try to regulate their labile emotional balance by excessive sports, sexual behavior, or sometimes impulsive aggressive behavior ('fight or flight'). Patients with borderline personality disorder (majority female, often with post-traumatic stress symptoms), on the other hand, tend to slide into 'freezing behavior' or 'dissociative states' when stressed emotionally. The self-injurious cutting or burning behavior is then used to put an end to these states of tension.

Given these considerations and positive clinical experience with dialectical behavior therapy (DBT) in patients with both ADHD and borderline personality disorder, it seemed a promising approach to offer certain elements of DBT skills training [23, 27] to patients with only ADHD.

The general approach of DBT concerns a form of therapy based on a principle driven approach with the two modes single and group therapy. A manualized 'skill training' [23, 27] comprising a number of modules is available for the group therapy, and this deals with coping with specific problem behavior.

In view of the ADHD symptomatic, the following assignment of modules for skill training of the DBT appeared appropriate:

Attention and concentration deficits ↔ 'Mindfulness'
Hyperactivity and Impulse control ↔ 'Distress tolerance'
Affective Instability ↔ 'Emotion regulation'
Interpersonal problems ↔ 'Interpersonal effectiveness'

Presentation of the Therapy Program
The following therapy elements were integrated as described (for an overview, see table 1).

Clarification
Patients with ADHD often do not recognize their problems as a symptom of a 'disorder'. Frequently being misdiagnosed, they feel together with other patients misunderstood in therapies and stop attending. A correct diagnosis alone often results in substantial relief since it allows the patients to understand their problems and symptoms as part of a recognized disorder. In order to prepare the patients in advance and to avoid premature termination of the therapy, they receive written information about their diagnosis of ADHD and the precise goals and sequence of the course of the therapy.

In the first session, following a general introduction, patients were educated regarding the symptoms and signs of ADHD. A general agreement is settled regarding the modalities of the therapy. Finally, the expectations and aims of the participants as well as possible limitations are discussed.

Table 1. Contents of the therapy – an overview

Clarification
Neurobiology/mindfulness I
Mindfulness II
Chaos and control
Dysfunctional behavior/behavior analysis I
Behavior analysis II
Emotion regulation
Depression/medication in ADHD
Impulse control
Stress management
Dependency
ADHD in relationship/self respect
Retrospect and outlook

Neurobiology/Mindfulness

Attention deficit is one of the primary deficits in ADHD. Many other symptoms derive from it. In the second section, patients are educated about the scientific knowledge regarding psychological aspects of attention and concentration and neurobiology of ADHD. Subsequently, the concept of mindfulness is discussed and patients are familiarized with training of mindfulness [23, 27]. Mindfulness skills are central to DBT. They are seen as psychological and behavioral versions of meditation skills 'drawn most heavily from the practice of Zen'. In DBT there are three 'what' skills (observing, describing, participating) and three 'how' skills (taking a non-judgmental stance, focusing on one thing at a time, being effective). In all following sessions, patients are asked to train these mindfulness skills and to repeat them on a daily basis as homework.

Chaos and Control

Disorganized behavior is one of the core diagnostic criteria of ADHD often resulting in difficulties at school, work and in interpersonal relationships. In the therapeutic context chaos is defined as follows: 'Chaos is, if ADHD takes control of me'. Control was defined as an antipodal concept: 'Control is, when I seize control of ADHD'. Following Hallowell and Ratey [9], a list of concrete advice (how to plan a day, how to organize help, etc.) are presented to the patients. Mechanisms how to precisely realize these suggestions in everyday life are discussed.

Dysfunctional Behavior/Behavior Analysis

Different behavior patterns are analyzed in this section. Dysfunctional behavior is defined as the kind of behavior patients want to change. The core concepts of behavior analysis (detailed and precise description of the behavior, preceding events, predisposing constellations, consequences, development of alternative strategies, prevention, apology, compensation) are introduced and taught to provide the patients with strategies for independent behavior analysis. Time and again, accurate examples of behavior analyses are practiced in the following group sessions.

Emotions

Emotional instability and brief recurrent depressive or dysphoric states or feelings of emptiness are all common in ADHD. In the section 'emotions', the patients are first informed about modern theories of emotion (primary emotions, signal and communicatory aspects of emotions, relationship cognition-emotion and emotion-behavior). Following this, exercises of emotional analysis (emotional record, emotional diary) and emotional regulation skills are demonstrated [23, 27].

Depression/Medication in ADHD

Patients are taught about the diagnosis and therapy of depressive disorders, since depression is very common in ADHD. Then, the principles of medical treatment of depression and ADHD are explained and every patient has the opportunity to report and discuss his personal experiences with medication.

Impulse Control

Impulse control and loss of impulse control are further core symptoms of ADHD. The exercises focusing on impulse control starts with behavior analyses of situations where loss of impulse control generally occurs frequently. The most common symptom reported is difficulty in controlling anger. Short- and long-term consequences of impulsive behavior are discussed and goal-directed behavior is trained [23, 27].

Stress

As mentioned above, disorganized behavior is another core symptom of ADHD. Affected patients often feel that this behavior is a result of emotional stress and experience this deficit as stressful in itself. Problems with planning and organizing sequential behavior often result in a situation in which patients with ADHD do several different things at the same time, feel pressurized, and end up finishing none of their projects.

The session focusing on this problem starts with education by informing the patients about the stress-performance relation. Subsequently, stress management techniques are trained, which are adapted according to personal resources. Exercises to improve personal stress tolerance are practiced.

Dependency

Substance abuse is one of the most common comorbid diagnoses in ADHD. Most patients suffering from ADHD have a history of drug abuse. To start dealing with this problem, patients are educated about symptoms and signs of dependency, effects and side effects of psychotropic substances in ADHD, and the nature and consequences of high risk and dependent behaviors often seen in ADHD (sexuality, high-risk sport, internet, etc.). Behavior analyses are then performed that focus on dependent behavior and define the aim of developing alternative behavioral strategies.

ADHD in Relationships/Self-Respect

The symptoms associated with ADHD render affected patients vulnerable to negative experiences during childhood, at school, university and work. In particular, the attention deficit is the reason why many patients do not achieve positions in private or professional life which correspond to their abilities and intelligence. Furthermore, the interpersonal relationships are affected at home and at work commonly resulting in criticism and rejection. This often leads to dramatically reduced self-esteem. The effects and consequences of ADHD including possible advantages of the disorder for the individual biography are discussed and patients have the opportunity to share their experiences.

Session with Partners and Family Members

Many families, partnerships and marriages are affected by the symptoms of ADHD of a family member or partner. Hallowell and Ratey [9] vividly describe the problems that often result from ADHD within interpersonal relationships. To address this problem, educational literature about ADHD as well as the content and the objectives of the psychotherapy is handed out to partners and family members. Arrangements are made to meet with partners or families of every participant separately. In these sessions, patients and partners have the opportunity to present and discuss their specific problems and coping strategies.

Retrospect and Outlook

In the last session the experiences in the therapy are summarized and the next steps are planned (e.g. transformation to a self-help group).

Structural Features

The following structural features have proven practical and helpful in carrying out group therapy with adults with ADHD:

Group Size

The optimal group size is 6–10 participants. No experience has been gained of groups exceeding 10 participants.

Duration

The duration of the program is originally designed to be around 13 sessions. These take place in a weekly cycle. The participants are informed that the diagnosis, preparation phase, and the possible consultations with relatives or partners will amount to a total duration of roughly 15–16 weeks.

Frequency

One 2-hour session per week. Early evening appointments have proven to be most convenient, enabling those working to participate in the group.

Structure of the Session

The weekly sessions are divided into two sections. In the first section the homework is discussed. Furthermore, the basic elements and instruments such as 'exercising mindfulness' and 'behavioral analysis' are the continuous subject of discussion and exercised.

The second section of the session is used for communicating new content. Roughly halfway through this section a 15- to 20-min break is recommended. Performing a short mindfulness exercise at the beginning of every section has proven to be a valuable ritual.

If possible, the groups should be under the guidance of two therapists. This is beneficial because it (1) reduces the chance of disturbing the regularity of the therapeutic sessions through absence or illness, and (2) it is easier to allocate the basic elements of the therapy to two therapists in the sense of seeking to establishing a balance between acceptance and change. One therapist can adopt with greater emphasis the aspect of acceptance, while the other tends more to embody the aspect of change. This approach should always be delivered in a balanced way whenever a distinct polarization emerges in the course of a group therapy.

Open or Closed Groups?

Given the structure of the program it is more appropriate to carry out the group therapy in a closed group.

Therapy Contract

Before proceeding with treatment the matter of formulating a written therapy contract should be discussed. The contract should set down clear rules about the conditions of participation and make clear the necessity for homework after the first session.

Homework

It has proven practical to indicate in the preparatory discussions and prior to the beginning of group therapy the effort involved in and importance of the homework, and to point out that repeated failure to complete the homework will be discussed as therapy interfering behavior

Dealing with Therapy Interfering Behavior

Therapy interfering behavior refers to the behavior of participants or therapists that makes execution of the therapy difficult or impossible for the participant, for the other participants, or for the therapist. Examples of such behavior are: unexcused absence, arriving late, omitting to do or finish homework, attending in an intoxicated state, aggressive behavior, and failure to observe acceptable personal limits of other participants or the therapist.

Therapy interfering behavior is always made a point of discussion when it represents appropriate topic of exercise relevant for the problems in daily life. For example, the issues of greater punctuality and regular participation will be discussed in detail at an early stage, presented as exemplary problems associated with ADHD, and worked on in behavioral analyses. When conducting a therapy it is therefore recommended that agreement is reached in the first session on the rules of punctuality and non-participation.

Conclusion

Despite the promising data on the effects of a disorder-oriented psychotherapy for ADHD in adults a number of issues remain to be resolved:

- Data on the long-term effect of psychotherapy is absent in most studies to date. Follow-up investigations are therefore necessary. One aspect of the disorder is that those affected are quicker and more enthusiastic to pick up on new ideas and suggestions. Particularly in interventions for ADHD it is especially important to verify the sustainability of changes.
- An important therapeutic variable of programs that are carried out in groups appears to be the group itself. It is therefore important to examine how much influence this 'group effect' has, that is, the experience made with those similarly affected of mutual understanding and coping, on the measured improvement in the symptomatic (individual versus group therapy).
- The possibility of implementing a disorder-oriented psychotherapy for ADHD under consideration of the different comorbidities is a largely unresolved issue. Clinical experience gives rise to two questions: (1) Which comorbidities in what intensity should be given priority and treated specifically because the primary ADHD therapy does not otherwise appear appropriate? (2) Are there disorders for which, in contrast, the treatment of ADHD should take place first or in parallel because the previous treatment approaches for those with comorbid ADHD result in a high non-responder rate.
- Which adult patients benefit from a medication-based therapy, which benefit from a psychotherapeutic approach, and in which is the combination of both of these most promising?
- Which modules should a disorder-oriented psychotherapy include and which modules can be omitted from the therapy programs developed to date (comparison of different therapeutic approaches)?

Despite these open questions, the implementation and further development of a disorder-oriented psychotherapy for ADHD in adults appears very promising, and the German Federal Ministry for Education and Research has therefore approved a large randomized multicenter study of 450 patients in a four-arm design (Methylphenidate vs. Psychotherapy following the Freiburg Treatment Program vs. Combination vs. Placebo) to investigate the effects of a 1-year treatment (intensive and maintenance treatment period), an investigation that also includes neurobiological variables (imaging-based measures and genetics) [21]. Follow-up examination of the persistent effects is also planned. The study is intended to make a further contribution to the differential therapeutic understanding of ADHD in adults and to closing the gap between our knowledge of ADHD in adults and that of ADHD in children and adolescents.

References

1 Nadeau KG: Life management skills for the adult with ADD; in Nadeau KG (ed): A Comprehensive Guide to Attention-Deficit Disorder in Adults: Research, Diagnosis, and Treatment. New York, Brunner/Mazel, 1995, pp 191–217.

2 McDermott SP: Cognitive therapy of adults with attention-deficit/hyperactive disorder; in Brown T (ed): Attention-Deficit Disorder and Comorbidities in Children, Adolescents, and Adults. Washington, American Psychiatric Press, 2000, pp 569–607.

3 Bemporad JR: Aspects of psychotherapy with adults with attention-deficit disorder; in Wasserstein J, Wolf LE, LeFever FF (eds): Adult Attention-Deficit Disorder – Brain Mechanisms and Life Outcomes. New York, The New York Academy of Sciences, 2001, pp 302–309.

4 Weiss MD, Weiss JR: A guide to the treatment of adults with ADHD. J Clin Psychiatry 2004;65(suppl 3):27–37.

5 Safren SA, Sprich S, Chulvick S, Otto MW: Psychosocial treatments for adults with attention-deficit/hyperactive disorder. Psychiatr Clin N Am 2004;27:349–360.

6 Murphy K: Psychosocial treatments for ADHD in teens and adults: a practice-friendly review. J Clin Psychol 2005;61:6007–6019.

7 Krause J, Ryffel-Rawak D: Therapie der Aufmerksamkeitsdefizit-/Hyperaktivitätsstörung im Erwachsenenalter. Psycho 2000;26:209–223.

8 Krause J: Psychodynamische Therapieansätze bei Erwachsenen mit ADHS. Psychotherapie 2008;13: 213–219.

9 Hallowell EM, Ratey J: Driven to Distraction. New York, Pantheon Books, 1994.

10 Hesslinger B, Tebartz van Elst L, Nyberg E, Dykierek P, Richter H, Ebert D: Psychotherapy of attention-deficit hyperactivity disorder in adults – a pilot study using a structured skills training program. Eur Arch Psychiatry Clin Neurosci 2002;252:177–184.

11 Stevenson CS, Whitmont S, Bornholt L, Livesy D, Stevenson RJ: A cognitive remediation program for adults with attention-deficit hyperactive disorder. Aust NZ J Psychiatry 2002;36:610–616.

12 Philipsen A, Richter H, Peters J, Alm B, Sobanski E, Colla M, Münzebrock M, Scheel C, Jacob C, Perlov E, Tebartz van Elst L, Hesslinger B: Structured group psychotherapy in adults with attention-deficit hyperactivity disorder – results of an open multicentre study. J Nerv Ment Dis 2007;195:1013–1019.

13 Zylowska L, Ackerman DL, Yang MH, Futrell JL, Horton NL, Hale TS, Pataki C, Smalley SL: Mindfulness meditation training in adults and adolescents with ADHD: a feasibility study. J Atten Disord 2008;11:737–746.

14 McDermott SP, Wilens TE: Cognitive-Behavioral Therapies: Treatment and Outcomes. Program of the American Psychiatric Association 2004 Annual Meeting, New York, 2004.

15 Safren SA, Perlman CA, Sprich S, Otto MW: Cognitive-behavioral therapy of ADHD in medication-treated adults with continued symptoms. Behav Res Ther 2005;43:831–842.

16 Rostain AL, Ramsay JR: A combined treatment approach for adults with ADHD – results of an open study of 43 patients. J Atten Disord 2006;10:150–159.

17 Weiss M, Hechtman L: Relationship between symptomatic and functional improvement in adult ADHD. Program and abstracts of the American Psychiatric Association 2005 Annual Meeting, Atlanta, 2005.

18 Bramham J, Young S, Bickerdike A, Spain D, McCartan D, Xenitidis K: Evaluation of group cognitive behavioral therapy for adults with ADHD. J Atten Disord 2008;12:434–441.
19 D'Amelio R, Retz W, Philipsen A, Rösler M: Psychoeducation and coaching in adult ADHD; in Manual for Leading Groups with Patients and Family Members (in German). Munich, Urban & Fischer, 2008.
20 Hesslinger B, Philipsen A, Harald R, Ebert D: Psychotherapy in Adult ADHD – A Workbook (in German). Göttingen, Hogrefe, 2004.
21 Philipsen A, van Elst LT, Lesch KP, Jans T, Warnke A: Effects and mechanisms of psychotherapy in the treatment of attention-deficit hyperactivity disorder (ADHD) in children and adults (in German). Psychother Psychosom Med Psychol 2009;59:132–140.
22 Grawe K: Psychologische Therapie. Göttingen, Hogrefe, 1998.
23 Linehan M: Cognitive-Behavioral Treatment of Borderline Personality Disorder. New York, The Guilford Press, 1993.
24 Philipsen A: Differential diagnosis and comorbidity of attention-deficit/hyperactivity disorder and borderline personality disorder in adults. Eur Arch Psychiatry Clin Neurosci 2006;256:i42–i46.
25 Philipsen A, Feige B, Hesslinger B, Scheel C, Ebert D, Limberger MF, Kleindienst N, Bohus M, Lieb K: Borderline typical symptoms in adult patients with attention-deficit/hyperactivity disorder. ADHD Attention Deficit Hyperactivity Disorders 2009 (in press).
26 Ceumern-Lindenstjerna I-A V, Brunner R, Parzer P, Fiedler P, Resch F: Borderline personality disorder and attentional biases. Theoretical models and empirical findings (in German). Fortschr Neurol Psychiat 2002;70:321–330.
27 Linehan M: Skills Training Manual for Treating Borderline Personality Disorder. New York, Guilford Press, 1993.

PD Dr. Alexandra Philipsen
Department of Psychiatry and Psychotherapy, University of Freiburg Medical School
Hauptstrasse 5
DE–79104 Freiburg (Germany)
Tel. +49 761 270 6501, Fax +49 761 270 6619, E-Mail alexandra.philipsen@uniklinik-freiburg.de

Retz W, Klein RG (eds): Attention-Deficit Hyperactivity Disorder (ADHD) in Adults.
Key Issues in Mental Health. Basel, Karger, 2010, vol 176, pp 174–186

Psychopharmacological Treatment of Attention-Deficit Hyperactivity Disorder in Adults

Götz-Erik Trott

Aschaffenburg, Germany

Abstract

Attention-deficit hyperactivity disorder (ADHD) in adults is a common disorder which results in a lot of secondary problems. Pharmacological treatment is essential in the management of ADHD. Stimulant treatment has for decades been proven to be effective and safe. Amphetamine was the first drug for this indication; most studies have been carried out with methylphenidate, which has been shown to be very effective and well tolerated. Newer extended-release methylphenidate preparations have considerable advantages. Because of hepatic side effects, pemoline no longer plays a role. Modafinil seems to have comparable effects like amphetamine. Atomoxetine is a potent norepinephrine-specific reuptake inhibitor which is approved for the treatment of ADHD in children, adolescents and adults. Tricyclic antidepressants may be third-line agents. Bupropion targets both ADHD and depressive symptoms which are frequent comorbid conditions. Clonidine and guanfacine have positive effects in patients with ADHD and comorbid tics. Several other compounds may be beneficial in ADHD treatment.

Attention-deficit hyperactivity disorder (ADHD) has been increasingly recognized as a chronic condition [1]. Already in the 1980s, Paul Wender [2] realized that ADHD patients remain in treatment also in early adulthood. Approximately one- to two-thirds of children with ADHD continue to manifest at least some clinically significant symptoms of the disorder into adulthood [3]. The symptom of hyperactivity shows best remission in adolescence, whereas impulsivity and inattention decline only slightly [4]. The prevalence of adult ADHD has been estimated in a recent study to be 4.4% [5].

There is common consent that untreated ADHD has a high risk of secondary problems in later life [6]. Studies in adults who have been diagnosed in childhood showed significantly higher rates of lower academic degrees, substance abuse and delinquency, impaired problems in occupational integration, more unwanted pregnancies, more children, more divorces and more contacts to medical services [7].

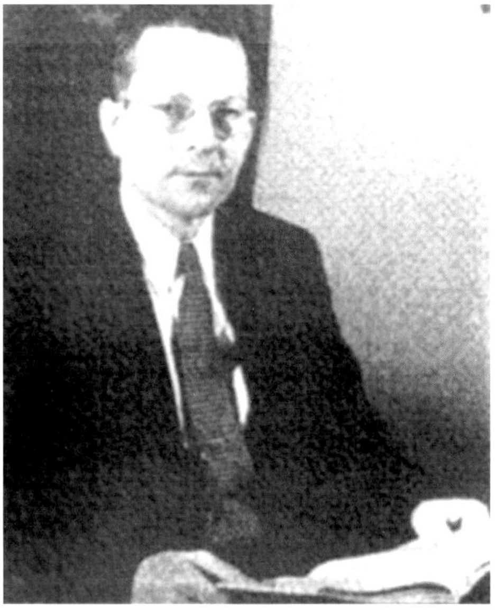

Fig. 1. Charles Bradley who in 1937 was the first to publish the beneficial effects of benzedrine in inattentive and restless children [8].

The beneficial effects of benzedrine in inattentive and restless children were first published by Charles Bradley in 1937 [8] (fig. 1). Lauretta Bender confirmed his findings [9], and in the 1960s, methylphenidate was introduced into the treatment of ADHD in children [10].

Stimulant medications are the first-line treatment options for the pharmacological treatment of ADHD. Methylphenidate is one of the best investigated drugs [11] which has been proven as being effective and safe in children, adolescents and in recent studies in adults [12–15]. In the Multimodal Treatment Study of ADHD (MTA) there were no significant differences between children receiving stimulant therapy alone and children receiving stimulant treatment with behavior therapy on ADHD outcome measures [16]. Although psychotherapeutic interventions can be beneficial in treating the broad sequelae of ADHD (e.g. low frustration tolerance, low self-esteem, poor social skills, etc.), stimulant medications are the most effective treatment for the target symptoms of inattention, hyperactivity and impulsivity [17, 18].

The primary goals of therapy should influence those symptoms that interfere most with the psychosocial functioning of the patient. So, treatment recommendations for the individual patient will greatly depend not only on the presence and severity of symptoms but also on the extent to which these symptoms impair functioning across different settings. The different drugs which have been shown to be effective in ADHD treatment enable the physician to realize a tailoring treatment of the individual patient.

Substances with proven benefit for adult ADHD treatment are stimulants, atomoxetine, several antidepressants and α-adrenergic agents (table 1).

Table 1. Substances in treatment of ADHD in adults

Stimulants			Atomoxetine	Antidepressants	Others
Pemoline	Amphetamine-based	Methylphenidate-based	Strattera®	Imipramine	Clonidine
Cylert®	Dexedrine®	Concerta®		Desipramine	Guanfacine
Tradon®	Adderall® Adderall XR® Vyvanse®	Daytrana® Medikinet retard® Metadate CD® Ritalin LA® Ritalin SR® Focalin®		Nortryptiline Buspiron Moclobemide	

Stimulants

Stimulant medications are the first-line treatment options for the pharmacological treatment of ADHD. As mentioned above, the efficacy of these substances was determined already in the 1930s. In 1944, the Swiss Leandro Panizzon developed methylphenidate [19] which is nowadays the most prescribed ADHD drug in the world.

Amphetamine-Based Stimulants

D-Amphetamine sulfate (Dexedrine®) is not available in all European countries. D-Isomer as well as L-isomer have pharmacological properties in ADHD – D-isomer 3–4 times more. Amphetamine releases dopamine from presynaptic neurons, it reaches peak plasma levels within 2–3 h with a plasma half-life between 4 and 6 h (but with substantial interindividual variability). The metabolization of dextroamphetamine occurs mainly in the liver, where deamination and *p*-hydroxylation transform it mainly to benzoic acid. A significant proportion is excreted in the urine, ranging from 2% in very alkaline urine to as high as 80% in very acid urine, so that high gastric activity and some drugs against urinary infections may affect concentration substantially. Behavioral effects are noticeable within 30–60 min after oral ingestion and usually dissipate within 4–6 h.

Adderall® is a combination of four dextroamphetamine/amphetamine salts, namely dextroamphetamine saccharate, amphetamine aspartate, dextroamphetamine sulfate and amphetamine sulfate. The extended-release preparation Adderall XR® uses a beaded delivery system and can be administered in sprinkle form – a beneficial effect was noted at 10–12 h in children [20]. Dexedrine® capsules have a half-life of about 10 h, but there is considerable variability in duration of effect among patients.

Vyvanse® (lisdexamfetamine dimesylate) is an inactive prodrug in which D-amphetamine is bonded to L-lysine, a naturally-occurring amino acid. It is designed as a capsule for once-a-day oral administration. Vyvanse® capsules are available with 20–70 mg of the compound. Lisdexamfetamine dimesylate remains inactive until converted and active D-amphetamine is gradually released. The T_{max} of lisdexamfetamine dimesylate is approximately 1 h. In studies with healthy adults with a history of stimulant abuse it tended to be less euphoric than D-amphetamine sulfate and had a later peak effect. The abuse liability and abuse potential of lisdexamfetamine dimesylate seems to be substantially less than D-amphetamine sulfate. It has a low potential for drug-drug interactions or inition of drug-drug interactions [21].

Adverse effects of stimulants can be caused by physiological effects of noradrenergic activation (increase of heart rate and blood pressure, contraction of bladder sphincter and bronchodilatation), those associated with pharmacokinetics of single or repeated doses waxing or waning over 3–4 h, different individual responses between doses and between two stimulants and other idiosyncratic responses. The most common side effects are loss of appetite, difficulties falling in sleep, headaches and stomachaches. In some predisposed patients, tics can occur. These side effects are generally mild, can be managed with adjustments of timing or dose and can be confirmed by interrupting medication. Adverse effects of stimulants are far less common and severe in controlled studies than their reputation in popular belief, opinion and prejudice. Dexamphetamine may theoretically predispose to slightly more noticeable side effects, especially to negative emotional symptoms [22]. A literature research revealed no information on the outcome of pregnancy in prescribed users of stimulants for ADHD [23]; as teratogenesis cannot be excluded, this problem should be considered in postpubertal and adult females.

Methylphenidate-Based Stimulants

Methylphenidate is the most extensively studied stimulant; it reaches plasma peak levels within 1.5–2.5 h after ingestion. The plasma half-life is usually between 2 and 3 h and the drug is entirely metabolized within 12–24 h, with almost none of the drug appearing in urine. The metabolic pathway for its decomposition and elimination seems to be via deesterification to ritalinic acid, to a lesser degree via hydroxylation to *p*-hydroxymethylphenidate, and the remainder to oxoritalinic acid and oxomethylphenidate, all of which are pharmacologically inactive. Behavioral effects occur within 30–60 min, with a peak within 1–3 h. It is important to note that interindividual variability exists with respect to these parameters. The plasma level does appear to be dose-related.

Immediate-release methylphenidate is the shortest acting stimulant medication option. Three times daily dosing is often required to maintain benefit throughout the day and patients may experience rebound of ADHD symptoms prior to the next dose as the medication wears off.

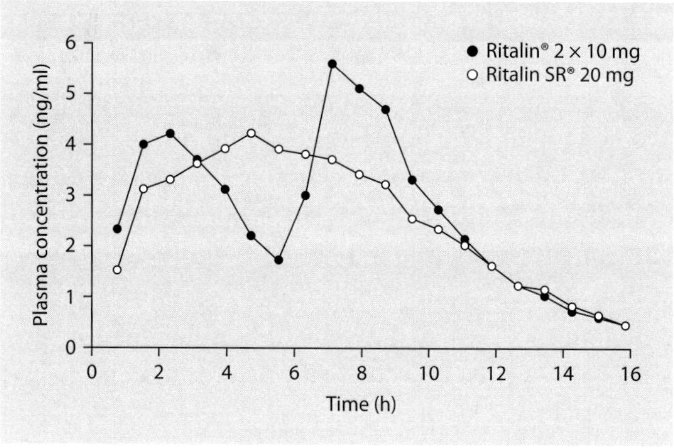

Fig. 2. Pharmacokinetics of Ritalin IR® vs. Ritalin SR® [adapted from 58].

A relatively new form of methylphenidate is the dextro isomer of methylphenidate dexmethylphenidate hydrochloride (Focalin®), which requires divided dosing (twice daily).

Methylphenidate sustained release (Ritalin SR®) was the first available form of long-acting methylphenidate. Although the sustained release form allowed in some patients the possibility of once-daily dosing, there was a delay in clinical effects and the peak effect varied for the individual patient (fig. 2).

The development of newer methylphenidate preparations with extended release expanded the options for longer acting coverage. Concerta® offers both immediate- and extended-release methylphenidate from the same capsule. An overcoat of the capsule provides the immediate release form within 30–60 min after administration. Then the osmotic pump delivery system (OROS®, i.e. osmotic-release oral system) releases methylphenidate gradually to allow for duration of effect of 10–12 h. The second peak level occurs at 6–8 h (fig. 3). The capsule cannot be chewed or crushed. Concerta® is available with 18, 36 and 54 mg, in the USA also with 72 mg. Concerta® is an effective dose-dependent treatment of ADHD in adults with a safety profile consistent with methylphenidate use in children and adults [24].

Metadate CD® (in Europe Equasym retard®) capsules contain a mixture of immediate- and delayed-release methylphenidate beads (Diffucaps) in a ratio of 3:7 (fig. 4). It is available in 10, 20 and 30 mg. The bioavailability and tolerability of Metadate CD® in adults is not altered when the capsule is opened and the beads are sprinkled on food [25].

Ritalin LA® (in France Ritalin LP®) uses the SODAS® (i.e. spheroidal oral drug absorption system) technology to integrate immediate and delayed release. The ratio of the two components is 1:1, so that less medication is delivered in the afternoon compared to Metadate CD® and Concerta®. Ritalin LA® is available in 20-, 30- and 40-mg capsules.

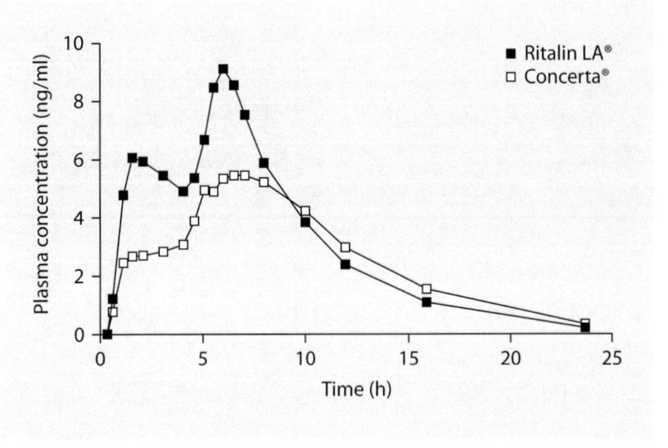

Fig. 3. Plasma concentration of Ritalin LA® 20 mg vs. Concerta® 18 mg [adapted from 58].

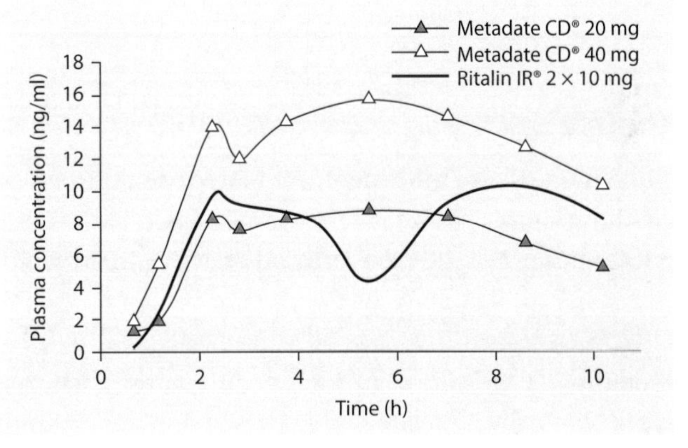

Fig. 4. Biphasic release of Metadate CD®/Equasym retard® vs. Ritalin IR® [adapted from 59].

Medikinet retard® is available only in Central Europe. The pellets contain methylphenidate in the ratio 1:1 immediate to delayed (after ca. 4 h) release. It is available in 5-, 10-, 20-, 30- and 40-mg preparations. A study with Medikinet retard® in adults with ADHD was carried out in Germany recently [15].

Daytrana® is a methylphenidate patch which should be worn 9 h; its effects continue for 3 h after it is removed. It is available in four patch sizes with 10, 15, 20 and 30 mg methylphenidate. The advantage of Daytrana® is the flexibility of managing the duration of the drug. It should be applied to the hip in the morning, and the patch provides medicine continuously. A daylong adhesion also during sport activities such as swimming, exercising and bathing is warranted.

Focalin XR® contains dexmethylphenidate hydrochloride, the active D-isomer of D,L-methylphenidate, and is available in four strengths, including 5-, 10- and 20-mg capsules. It has a bimodal release profile with ratio 1:1 and uses the SODAS®

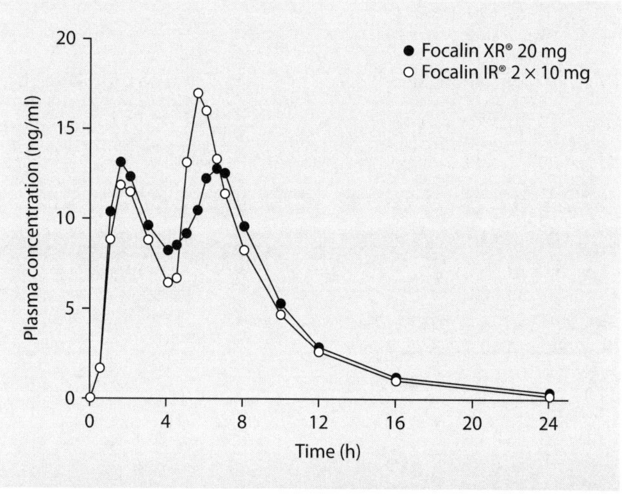

Fig. 5. Mean dexmethylphenidate plasma concentration [adapted from 60].

technology. The first peak concentration is reached in about 90 min after ingestion, the second one in about 6.5 h (fig. 5). A study in children showed that dexmethylphenidate hydrochloride is not better or safer than methylphenidate, but has a longer duration of action [26]. In a large controlled study, dexmethylphenidate-extended release has proven to be a safe and effective treatment for adults with ADHD [27].

Other Stimulants

Modafinil (Provigil®, Vigil®) has been approved for treatment of narcolepsy in adults. It is chemically unrelated to methylphenidate or amphetamine. Compared to these two substances it seems less likely to cause irritability and excitement. It appears to act on the frontal cortex and is more selective in its area of action than the traditional stimulants [28]. Modafinil improves in adults short memory span, visual memory, spatial planning and stop-signal motor inhibition [29]. In a randomized double-blind placebo-controlled study comparing the efficacy of modafinil to that of dextroamphetamine in adults, both medications were well tolerated and showed significant improvement [30]. The most common adverse events were insomnia, headache and decreased appetite; the severity of symptoms was mild to moderate. Modafinil may have advantages over current therapies for ADHD in that it can be administered once daily and has fewer reinforcing properties than traditional stimulants [31].

Pemoline (Cylert®, Tradon®) lacks significant sympathomimetic activity and can be administered once a day. It is usually started at a dose of 40 mg in the morning and then increased gradually by 20 mg/week to 0.5–3 mg/kg day. It takes about 1–2 h to take effect, lasts up to 8 h and it may take several days to build up to have an clinical effect. Because of increasing concerns about hepatotoxicity, biweekly liver function monitoring is required. Actually, pemoline is a third-line medication.

Second-Line Agents

Outside the psychostimulants, noradrenergic and dopaminergic active compounds including monoamine oxidase inhibitors [32, 33], secondary amine tricyclic antidepressants [34] and bupropion [35] have been found superior to placebo in controlled clinical studies. Possible advantages of these compounds over stimulants include a longer duration of action without symptom rebound, minimal risk of abuse and as the potential treatment of comorbid internalizing symptoms.

Tricyclic Antidepressants
One of the best established second-line treatments for ADHD are the tricyclic antidepressants (TCAs). Out of 33 studies evaluating TCAs in children, adolescents and adults, 91% reported positive effects on ADHD symptoms [36]. Imipramine and desipramine are the most studied TCAs. Although most TCA studies were relatively brief, lasting from a few weeks to several months, nine studies reported enduring effects for up to 2 years. The outcome in both short- and long-term studies were equally positive [37]. Desipramine at an average dose of 150 mg was statistically and clinically more effective than placebo in adults [38]. Similar to atomoxetine, tricyclics block the norepinephrine transporter, which is believed to attenuate ADHD symptoms by increasing norepinephrine in the synapse. Anticholinergic side effects have restricted clinical use of these drugs.

Atomoxetine
Atomoxetine is a potent norepinephrine-specific reuptake inhibitor that has been studied in over 1,800 children and over 250 adults [37, 39, 40]. In the USA, atomoxetine was approved in November 2002 for the treatment of ADHD in children, adolescents and adults. Atomoxetine does not appear to affect the dopamine systems as directly as the stimulants do, but causes a secondary increase in dopamine levels in the prefrontal cortex [41]. It is metabolized primarily via the cytochrome P450 (CYP) 2D6 enzymes in the liver, so that poor metabolizers need reduced target dosages. Dosing is recommended to be initiated at 0.5 mg/kg, with titration up to 1.2 mg/kg. A dose of atomoxetine is generally administered either once or twice daily. Possible side effects include decreased appetite, nausea/stomach upset, decreased sleep and a mild increase in pulse or blood pressure. Atomoxetine can lead to urinary retention and can cause problems with sexual functioning in some individuals. Atomoxetine ameliorates ADHD symptoms in adults, usually has no rebound effect like stimulants, and improves their perceived quality of life [42, 43]. Atomoxetine has a slower onset to action than stimulants do; thus effects may not be seen until the end of the first week of treatment.

Bupropion
Bupropion hydrochloride (Wellbutrin®, Zyban®) is an aminoketone antidepressant that has been used to treat ADHD. Unique advantages of using this drug are that it

may target both ADHD and depressive symptoms and the possibility of once-daily dosing and 24 h coverage. In studies, bupropion has shown modest efficacy in ADHD treatment in adults [44]. Although bupropion is well tolerated by most patients, in rare cases it induces seizures, which is why the drug should not be given to patients with a history of seizure disorders or bulimia. This substance is efficacious for controlling cigarette smoking which is increased in ADHD patients [45].

α_{2A}-Adrenoreceptor Agonist

Clonidine (Catapress®, Catapresan®) and guanfacine (Tenex®, Estulic®) have been used in adults for the treatment of hypertension. These substances have shown positive effects in ADHD patients, especially for those with tics, impulsivity and aggression rather than with inattention. The sedating property can cause problems concentrating on work and traffic. Besides this, α-adrenergic agents may also cause decreased pulse and blood pressure, as well as dry mouth, depression and confusion.

Clonidine is not known to have long-term adverse effects. It is a relatively short-acting compound with plasma half-life ranging from approximately 5.5 h in children to 8.5 h in adults. Daily doses should be titrated and individualized. A usual daily dose ranges from 3 to 10 μg/kg given generally in divided doses 2–4 times a day. Therapy is usually initiated at the lowest manufactured dose of a half tablet and increased depending on clinical response and adverse effects. A meta-analysis of 39 studies investigating the use of clonidine in ADHD treatment indicated a moderate effect size, with particular benefit for children with comorbid conduct disorder, developmental delay and tic disorder [46].

The more selective α_{2A}-agonist guanfacine *(Tenex®, Estulic®)* may have a similar spectrum of benefits to those of clonidine with less sedation and longer duration of action. The usual daily dose of guanfacine ranges from 40 to 85 μg/kg, given generally in divided doses, 2–3 times a day. In a study in adults with ADHD, guanfacine was shown to improve both ADHD symptoms and a cognitive test of response inhibition as measured by the Stroop [47].

Other Compounds

Venlafaxine (Effexor®, Trevilor®) has shown to be helpful for some adults with ADHD. In an open study a significant reduction in ADHD symptomatology was described; it was well tolerated and most patients experienced only mild side effects [48, 49]. As comedication with stimulants, venlafaxine seems to be superior to other antidepressants in the treatment of ADHD and comorbid social phobia or depression.

An open-label study suggests that the NMDA receptor antagonist memantine may be a safe and possible effective treatment of ADHD in pediatric patients [50].

There are only a few experiences of estrogen supplementation in females with ADHD. Some women report that their ADHD symptoms worsen during the premenstrual period and during the perimenopausal years and improvement in memory and attention span after estrogen supplementation. Since estrogen affects many systems in the body, the risks and benefits should be considered. More systematic research is needed to clear the relation between ADHD and estrogen.

Nicotine enhances dopaminergic neurotransmission, and poor regulation of the nicotinergic receptors may be involved in the pathophysiology of ADHD. A transdermal nicotine patch seems to improve some symptoms of ADHD [51, 52].

A few studies show correlations of zinc level with either clinical severity or a change thereof in response to stimulant or chemical challenge [53]. The possible role of zinc in ADHD is not yet clear, but there is strong evidence to warrant further controlled studies in well-diagnosed samples [54].

Conclusions

ADHD in adults is a chronic condition which requires efficient therapy to reduce impairing symptoms. Non-pharmacologic interventions tested in children and adolescents were not more effective than medication in treatment of the core symptoms of ADHD [55]. There is evidence that the situation in adults does not differ from children and adolescents. Long-standing clinical experience dictates that coaching and problem-based and solution-oriented counseling of the patient and his family are valuable and necessary adjuncts to drug therapy.

First-line pharmacotherapies include the FDA-approved medications. There is the longest experience with stimulants. Both amphetamine and methylphenidate have a history of more than 40 years of robust response, good tolerability and safety. In controlled studies, methylphenidate has demonstrated the efficacy and tolerability in adults [12–15]. The different longer acting stimulants enable the physician to practice a tailoring treatment with the individual patient. The cost-effectiveness relation of these compounds is very good [56, 57].

Atomoxetine is a non-stimulant ADHD medication which has proven efficacy in adults. At this time there are no adequately powered head-to-head studies and thus no rational guidelines inform the relative position of this drug in the group of anti-ADHD treatments. Actually, atomoxetine is indicated for conditions in which tics, poor response to stimulants or side effects and certain comorbidities like depression and anxiety are present.

Before prescribing medication it is essential to apply a careful differential diagnosis in the assessment of the ADHD patient that considers psychiatric, social, cognitive, educational, occupational and medical/neurological factors. Realistic expectations of the treatment, definitions of target symptoms and careful assessment of the potential risks and benefits of each kind of intervention are required.

References

1 Trott GE: Attention-deficit/hyperactivity disorder in the course of life. Eur Arch Psychiatry Clin Neurosci 2006;256(suppl 1):21–25.

2 Wender PH, Reimherr FW, Wood DR: A controlled study of methylphenidate in the treatment of attention-deficit disorder residual type in adults. Am J Psychiatry 1985;142:547–552.

3 Barkley RA: Attention-Deficit/Hyperactivity Disorder: A Handbook for Diagnosis and Treatment, ed 2. New York, Guilford Press, 1998.

4 Biederman J, Mick E, Faraone SV: Age-dependent decline of attention-deficit hyperactivity disorder. Am J Psychiatry 2000;157:816–818.

5 Kessler RC, Ader L, Barkley R, Biederman J, Conners CK, Demler O, Faraone SV, Greenhill LL, Howes MJ, Secnik K, Spencer T, Ustun TB, Walters EE, Zaslavsky AM: The prevalence and correlates of adult ADHD in the United States: results from the national comorbidity survey replication. Am J Psychiatry 2006;163:716–723.

6 Taylor E, Chadwick O, Heptinstall E, Danckaerts M: Hyperactivity and conduct problems as a risk factor for adolescent development. J Am Acad Child Adolesc Psychiatry 1996;35:1213–1226.

7 Barkley RA, Fischer M, Smallish L Fletcher K: The persistence of attention-deficit/hyperactivity disorder into young adulthood as a function of reporting source and definition of disorder. J Abnorm Psychol 2002;111:279–289.

8 Bradley C: The behavior of children receiving benzedrine. Am J Psychiatry 1937;94:577–585.

9 Bender L, Cottington F: The use of amphetamine sulfate (benzedrine) in child psychiatry. Am J Psychiatry 1942;99:116–121.

10 Eisenberg L: The management of the hyperkinetic child. Dev Med Child Neurol 1966;8:593–598.

11 Spencer T, Biederman J, Wilens T, Harding M, O'Donnell D, Griffin S: Pharmacotherapy of attention-deficit/hyperactivity disorder across the life cycle. J Am Acad Child Adolesc Psychiatry 1996; 35:1460–1469.

12 Faraone SV, Spencer T, Aleardi M, Pagano C, Biederman J: Meta-analysis of the efficacy of methylphenidate for treating adult attention-deficit/hyperactivity disorder. J Clin Psychopharmacology 2004;24:24–29.

13 Kösters M, Becker T, Kilian R, Fegert JM, Weinmann S: Limits of meta-analysis: methylphenidate in the treatment of adult attention-deficit hyperactivity disorder. J Psychopharmacol (2008); Online First DOI: 10.1177/0269881108092338.

14 Spencer T, Biederman J, Wilens T, Doyle R, Surman C, Prince J, Mick E, Aleardi M, Herzig K, Faraone S: A large, double-blind, randomized clinical trial of methylphenidate in the treatment of adults with attention-deficit/hyperactivity disorder. Biol Psychiatry 2005;57:456–463.

15 Rösler M, Fischer R, Ammer R, Ose C, Retz W, on behalf of the study group: a randomised, placebo-controlled, 24-week, study of low-dose extended-release methylphenidate in adults with attention-deficit/hyperactivity disorder. Eur Arch Psychiatry Clin Neurosci 2009;259:120–129.

16 MTA Cooperative Group: A 14-month randomized clinical trial of treatment strategies for attention-deficit/hyperactivity disorder. Arch Gen Psychiatry 1999;56:1073–1086.

17 Jensen PS; Hinshaw SP, Kraemer HC: ADHD comorbidity findings from the MTA study: comparing comorbid subgroups. J Am Acad Child Adolesc Psychiatry 2001;40:147–158.

18 Foster EM, Jensen PS, Schlander M, Pelham WE, Hechtman L, Arnold LE, Swanson JM, Wigal T: Treatment for ADHD: is more complex treatment cost-effective for more complex cases? Health Serv Res 2007;42:165–182.

19 Panizzon L: La preparazione di pridile peperidilarilaceto-nitrile e di alcuni prodotti di trasformazione. Helv Chim Acta 1944;27:1748–1756.

20 Kutcher S: Practitioner review: the pharmacotherapy of adolescent depression. J Child Psychol Psychiatry 1997;38:755–767.

21 Krishnan S, Moncrief S: An evaluation of the cytochrome P450 inhibition potential of lisdexamfetamine in human liver microsomes. Drug Metab Dispos 2007;35:1:180–184.

22 Efron D, Jarman FC, Barker M: 'Side effects' of methylphenidate and dexamphetamine in children with attention-defi cit hyperactivity disorder: a double-blind crossover trial. Pediatrics 1997;100:662–666.

23 Ashton H, Gallagher P, Moore B: The adult psychiatrist's dilemma: psychostimulant use in attention-deficit/hyperactivitydisorder. J Psychopharmacology 2006;20:602–610.

24 Medori R, Ramos-Quiroga JA, Casas M, Kooij JJ, Niemelä A, Trott GE, Lee E, Buitelaar JK: A randomized, placebo-controlled trial of three fixed dosages of prolonged-release OROS methylphenidate in adults with attention-deficit/hyperactivity disorder. Biol Psychiatry 2008;63:981–989.

25 Pentikis HS, Simmons RD, Benedict MF, Hatch SJ: Methylphenidate bioavailability in adults when an extended-release multiparticulate formulation is administered sprinkled on food or as an intact capsule. J Am Acad Child Adolesc Psychiatry 2002;41: 443–449.
26 Wigal S, Swanson JM, Feifel D, Sangal RB, Elia J, Casat CD, Zeldis JB, Conners CK: A double-blind, placebo-controlled trial of dexmethylphenidate hydrochloride and D,L-threomethylphenidate in children with attention-deficit/hyperactivity disorder. J Am Acad Child Adolesc Psychiatry 2004;43: 1406–1414.
27 Spencer TJ, Adler LA, McGough JJ, Muniz R, Jiang H, Pestreich L, Adult ADHD Research Group: Efficacy and safety of dexmethylphenidate-extended release capsules in adults with attention-deficit/hyperactivity disorder. Biol Psychiatry 2007;61: 1380–1387.
28 Ballon JS, Feifel D: A systematic review of modafinil: potential clinical uses and mechanisms of action. J Clin Psychiatry 2006;67:727–735.
29 Turner DC, Clark L, Dowson J, Robbins TW, Sahakian BJ: Modafinil improves cognition and response in adult attention-deficit/hyperactivity disorder. Biol Psychiatry 2004;55:10:1031–1040.
30 Taylor FB, Russo J: Efficacy of modafinil compared to dextroamphetamine for the treatment of attention-deficit hyperactivity disorder in adults. J Child Adolesc Psychopharmacol 2000;10:311–320.
31 Turner DC: A review of the use of modafinil for attention-deficit hyperactivity disorder. Expert Rev Neurother 2006;6:455–468.
32 Zametkin AJ, Rapoport JL, Murphy DL, Linnoila M, Ismond D: Treatment of hyperactive children with monoamine oxidase inhibitors. Arch Gen Psychiatry 1985;42:962–966.
33 Trott GE, Friese HJ, Menzel M, Nissen G: Use of moclobemide in children with attention-deficit hyperactivity disorder. Psychopharmacology 1992; 106(suppl 1):134–136.
34 Wilens TE, Biederman J, Geist DE, Steingard R, Spencer T: Nortryptiline in the treatment of attention-deficit hyperactivity disorder: a chart review. J Am Acad Child Adolesc Psychiatry 1993;32:343–349.
35 Conners K, Casat C, Gualtieri T, Weller E, Reader M, Reiss A, Weller R, Khayrallah M, Ascer J: Bupropion hydrochloride in attention-deficit disorder with hyperactivity. J Am Acad Child Adolesc Psychiatry 1996;35:1314–1321.
36 Spencer T, Biederman J, Wilens T: Pharmacotherapy of ADHD: a lifespan perspective; in Oldham J, Riba M (eds): American Psychiatric Press Review of Psychiatry. Washington, American Psychiatric Press, 1997, pp 87–128.
37 Biederman J, Spencer T, Wilens T: Evidence-based pharmacotherapy for attention-deficit hyperactivity disorder. Int J Neuropsychopharmacol 2004;7:77–97.
38 Wilens TE, Biederman J, Prince J, Spencer TJ, Faraone SV, Warburton R, Schleifer D, Harding M, Linehan C, Geller D: Six week double-blind placebo-controlled study of desipramine for adult attention-deficit hyperactivity disorder. Am J Psychiatry 1996;153:1147–1153.
39 Michelson D, Adler L, Spencer T, Reimherr FW, West SA, Allen AJ, Kelsey D, Wernicke J, Dietrich A, Milton D: Atomoxetine in adults with ADHD: two randomized, placebo-controlled studies. Biol Psychiatry 2003;53:112–120.
40 Adler LA, Spencer T, Brown TE, Holdnack J, Saylor K, Schuh K, Trzepacz PT, Williams DW, Kelsey D: Once-daily atomoxetine for adult attention-deficit/hyperactivity disorder: a 6-month, double-blind trial. J Clin Psychopharmacol 2009;29:44–50
41 Stahl SM: Neurotransmission of cognition. 1. Dopamine is a hitchhiker in frontal cortex: norepinephrine transporters regulate dopamine. J Clin Psychiatry 2003;64:4–5.
42 Adler LA, Sutton VK, Moore RJ, Dietrich AP, Reimherr FW, Sangal RB, Sylor KE, Secnik K, Kelsey DK, Allen AJ: Quality of life assessment in adult patients with attention-deficit/hyperactivity disorder treated with atomoxetine. J Clin Psychopharmacol 2006;26:648–652.
43 Faraone SV, Biederman J, Spencer T, Michelson D, Adler L, Reimherr F, Glatt SJ: Efficacy of atomoxetine in adult attention-deficit/hyperactivity disorder: a drug-placebo response curve analysis. Behav Brain Funct 2005;3:16.
44 Wilens T, Haight BR, Horrigan JP, Hudziak JJ, Rosenthal NE, Connor DF, Hampton KD, Richard NE: Bupropion XL in adults with ADHD: a randomized placebo-controlled study. Biol Psychiatry 2005;57:793–801.
45 Krause KH, Dresel SH, Krause J, Kung HF, Tatsch K, Ackenheil M: Stimulant like action of nicotine on striatal dopamine transporter in the brain of adults with attention-deficit hyperactivity disorder. Int J Neuropsychopharmacol 2002;5:111–113.
46 Connor DF, Fletcher KE, Swanson JM: A meta-analysis of clonidine for symptoms of attention-deficit hyperactivity disorder. J Am Acad Child Adolesc Psychiatry 1999;38:1551–1559.
47 Taylor FB: Comparing guanfacine and dextroamphetamine for adult ADHD: efficacy and implications. 153rd Annual Meeting of the American Psychiatric Association, Chicago 2000.

48 Findling RL, Schwartz MA, Flannery DJ, Manos MJ: Venlafaxine in adults with attention-deficit/hyperactivity disorder: an open clinical trial. J Clin Psychiatry 1996;57:184–189.
49 Krause KH, Dresel S, Krause J: Neurobiologie der Aufmerksamkeitsdefizit-/Hyperaktivitätsstörung. Psychoneuro 2002;26:199–208.
50 Findling RL, McNamara NK, Stransbrey RJ, Maxhimer R, Periclou A, Mann A, Graham SM: A pilot evaluation on the safety, tolerability, pharmacokinetics, and effectiveness of memantine in pediatric patients with attention-deficit/hyperactivity disorder combined type. J Child Adolesc Psychopharmacol 2007;17:19–33.
51 Gehricke JG, Whalen CK, Jamner LD, Wigal TL, Steinhoff K: The reinforcing effects of nicotine and stimulant medication in the everyday lives of adult smokers with ADHD: a preliminary examination. Nicotine Tob Res 2006;8:37–47.
52 Poltavski DV, Petros T: Effects of transdermal nicotine on attention in adult non-smokers with and without attentional deficits. Physiol Behav 2006;87: 614–624.
53 Krause KH, Krause J: Dopamintransporter – Struktur, Funktion und Bedeutung für die ADHS. Psychoneuro 2006;32:209–214.
54 Arnold LE, DiSilvestro RA: Zinc in attention-deficit/hyperactivity disorder. J Child Adolesc Psychopharmacol 2005;15:619–627.
55 Brown RT, Amler RW, Freeman WS, Perrin JM, Stein MT, Feldman HM, Pierce K, Wolraich ML: Treatment of attention-deficit/hyperactivity disorder: overview of the evidence. Pediatrics 2005;115: 749–757.
56 Jensen PS, Garcia JA; Glied S, Crowe M, Foster EM, Schlander M, the MTA Cooperative Group: Cost-effectiveness of ADHD treatments: findings from the MTA study. Am J Psychiatry 2005;162:1628–1636
57 Schlander M: Long-acting medications for the hyperkinetic disorders: a note on cost-effectiveness. Eur Child Adolesc Psychiatry 2007;16:421–429.
58 Markowitz JS, Straughn AB, Patrick KS, DeVane CL, Pestreich L, Lee J, Wang Y, Muniz R: Pharmacokinetics of methylphenidate after oral administration of two modified-release formulations in healthy adults. Clin Pharmacokinet 2003;42:393–401.
59 Wigal SB, Sanchez DY, DeCory HH, D'Imperio JM, Swanson JM: Selection of the optimal dose ratio for a controlled-delivery formulation of methylphenidate. J Appl Res 2003;3:46–63.
60 www.fda.gov/medwatch/safety/2006/Apr_PIs/FocalinXR_PI.pdf

Prof. Götz-Erik Trott, MD
Luitpoldstrasse 2–4
DE–63739 Aschaffenburg (Germany)
Tel. +49 6021 32 54 53, Fax +49 6021 32 54 51, E-Mail praxis-trott@t-online.de

Author Index

Subject Index